LIFE–DEATH DECISIONS IN HEALTH CARE

SERIES IN DEATH EDUCATION, AGING, AND HEALTH CARE
HANNELORE WASS, CONSULTING EDITOR

ADVISORY BOARD
Herman Feifel, Ph.D.
Jeanne Quint Benoliel, R.N., Ph.D.
Balfour Mount, M.D.

Benoliel	Death Education for the Health Professional
Davidson	The Hospice: Development and Administration, Second Edition
Degner, Beaton	Life–Death Decision Making in Health Care
Doty	Effective Communication and Assertion for Older Persons
Epting, Neimeyer	Personal Meanings of Death: Applications of Personal Construct Theory to Clinical Practice
Stillion	Death and the Sexes: A Differential Examination of Longevity, Attitudes, Behaviors, and Coping Skills
Turnbull	Terminal Care
Vachon	Occupational Stress in the Care of the Critically Ill, the Dying, and the Bereaved
Wass	Dying: Facing the Facts
Wass, Corr	Childhood and Death
Wass, Corr	Helping Children Cope with Death: Guidelines and Resources, Second Edition
Wass, Corr, Pacholski, Forfar	Death Education II: An Annotated Resource Guide
Wass, Corr, Pacholski, Sanders	Death Education: An Annotated Resource Guide

IN PREPARATION

Curran	Adolescent Suicide
Haber	Long-Term Health Care Alternatives for the Elderly
Lonetto	Explaining Death and Dying
Riker	Retirement Counseling: A Handbook for Action
Stillion	Innovative Therapies in the Care of the Terminally Ill, the Dying, and the Bereaved
Stillion, McDowell, May	Suicide Across the Lifespan: Premature Exits
Wass, Berardo, Neimeyer	Dying: Facing the Facts, Second Edition

LIFE–DEATH
DECISIONS
IN HEALTH CARE

Lesley F. Degner
Manitoba Nursing Research Institute
School of Nursing, University of Manitoba

Janet I. Beaton
Graduate Program in Nursing
School of Nursing, University of Manitoba

● HEMISPHERE PUBLISHING CORPORATION, Washington
A subsidiary of Harper & Row, Publishers, Inc.

Cambridge   New York   Philadelphia   San Francisco
London   Mexico City   São Paulo   Singapore   Sydney

1 2 3 4 5 6 7 8 9 0   B R B R   8 9 8 7

This book was set in Press Roman by Hemisphere Publishing Corporation. The editors were Christine Flint Lowry and Elizabeth Maggiora; the production supervisor was Miriam Gonzalez; and the typesetter was Rita Shapiro.
Braun-Brumfield, Inc. was printer and binder.

Library of Congress Cataloging-in-Publication Data

Degner, Lesley F., date.
    Life-death decisions in health care.

    (Series in death education, aging, and health care)
    Bibliography: p.
    Includes index.
    1. Medicine—Decision making. 2. Life and death, Power over—Decision making. I. Beaton, Janet I., date. II. Title, III. Series. [DNLM. 1. Decision Making. 2. Delivery of Health Care—Canada. 3. Life Support Care. 4. Terminal Care. W 84 DC2 D3L]
    R723.5.D4 1987 610 86-31818
    ISBN 0-89116-399-9
    ISSN 0275-3510

To all the patients, families and health professionals

whose willingness to share their experiences

made this book possible.

CONTENTS

PREFACE

What happens when treatment decisions are made for patients with life-threatening illnesses? This book focuses on how treatment decisions are made within the context of modern health care. The initial report on this topic was presented to our major funding agency, Health and Welfare Canada, in 1981. While we received positive feedback from our professional colleagues after publication of that report, it was the wide publicity received by the Dawson* case that made us realize our findings might be useful to a more general audience. As a result, we decided to convert our original report, which had been primarily intended for a scientific audience, into a book for a broader readership.

Here we examine life–death decisions from the perspective of patients, families, and health professionals. We describe what *does* happen when treatment decisions are made, rather than what *should* happen, and as a result, this book is *descriptive* rather than *prescriptive*. Our description is grounded in the realities of clinical practice, and is derived from events that occurred in the lives of real people.

In March 1983, the parents of Stephen Dawson, a severely retarded seven-year-old boy, refused consent for surgery to revise a blocked shunt in his brain. The child was apprehended by the family and child service of the province of British Columbia, which petitioned the Provincial Court to permit the surgery. The judge ordered the child to be returned to the custody of his parents, but a few days later the Supreme Court of British Columbia reversed the decision and ordered that the surgical procedure be carried out. Stephen Dawson subsequently had his shunt revised and remains alive at the time of this writing.

The book describes how treatment decisions are actually made when patients develop life-threatening conditions. It also describes the factors that influence decision making, and how the participants in the process are affected by their involvement in this difficult field of health care. Because our description was formulated from real incidents of clinical decision making, we are able to examine what happens when things go right, and what happens when things go wrong.

We would like to make it clear what this book is *not* about. It is not a book about death and dying, or grief and grieving, although these topics inevitably arise given the nature of our initial question. The book is not written exclusively from the perspective of health care consumers or health professionals, nor does it focus on specific age groups, disease entities, or treatment types. Rather, it represents an attempt to identify underlying commonalities. The book is not social criticism or a "how-to" manual. Our intent is to provide both health professionals and consumers with a better understanding of the dynamics of life–death decision making and its impact on participants.

This book will help both health professionals and consumers. For consumers, the book should answer a number of questions, the most important of which is: "How will decisions be made about my treatment should I become seriously ill?" Consumers can make sense of past experience since the text describes aspects of health care that are not ordinarily visible to patients and families. It will also acquaint consumers with the clinical realities facing health professionals who practice in this fast-moving and crisis-ridden area of health care.

The book provides health professionals with the opportunity to compare their clinical experiences with our general description. We recognize our discussion may challenge some commonly held assumptions, particularly assumptions about the ability of patients and families to participate in decision making. More importantly, the book provides health professionals with a language for categorizing their decision-making processes. The systematic application of this language in clinical practice could lead to more effective communication and less conflict both among health professionals, and between health professionals and their clients.

The experience of writing this book forced us to reexamine our original description of life–death decision making. On the basis of this new perspective, we formulated both general and specific recommendations that went far beyond those in our original report. We believe that the implementation of these recommendations could significantly improve the quality of health care for life-threatened patients and their families.

Lesley F. Degner
Janet I. Beaton

ACKNOWLEDGMENTS

The original funding for the research upon which this book is based was supplied by National Health Grant Number 607-1041-21, Health and Welfare, Canada. We are also indebted to the Rockefeller Foundation for the scholar-in-residence awards that permitted our collaboration on this book during April and May of 1984 at the Villa Serbelloni, and to the University of Manitoba Research Grants Committee for providing the travel funds that enabled us to assume these awards.

In any scholarly endeavor, there are always individuals whose contributions have a significant influence on the quality of the final product. Throughout the 10 years during which this project was initiated and brought to completion, we were fortunate to have as a friend and colleague, Dr. Helen Preston Glass. Her personal support of our research careers, and her thoughtful encouragement throughout this project, provide only one example of her life long commitment to the development of nursing research in Canada. In many ways, this book is a tribute to that commitment.

Our consultants, Dr. Jeanne Quint Benoliel and Dr. Anselm Strauss, provided invaluable assistance during data collection and analysis for the original study. Jeanne Benoliel has continued to provide encouragement for our work, and we are particularly grateful for this support. Her research into the effects of life-threatening illnesses on both patients and their caregivers has provided a standard of excellence for all nurse investigators.

We would like to recognize our fellow scholars at the Villa Serbelloni, whose warmth and friendship provided us with lasting memories of a very special experience. Our thanks also to Angela Barmettler, Roberto Celli, and their staff for their gracious hospitality.

Finally, we would like to thank our "coach," who kept the coffee coming during our last, frenetic week of writing at Minaki Lodge. As well, our Editor, Ed Unrau, for his many helpful suggestions; Kaaren Neufeld, for preparation of the final manuscript; our students and colleagues at the University of Manitoba School of Nursing; and our families, who over many years have so patiently endured our preoccupation with this project.

Lesley F. Degner
Janet I. Beaton

INTRODUCTION

Your husband has had a cardiac arrest.

The tumor was malignant.

Your baby has only a 50 percent chance of surviving.

This is the kind of bad news anyone dreads receiving. Words like "terminal," "poor prognosis," and "cancerous" bring with them an ominous chill when applied to people we know or care about. We become acutely aware of our own vulnerability, and that someday we too may be the recipients of bad news.

People diagnosed with a life-threatening illness are suddenly propelled, along with their families, into an unfamiliar environment. They must communicate with a confusing variety of health professionals; they are bombarded by an array of frightening and often physically distressing tests and treatments; and they are forced to alter almost every aspect of their day-to-day lives. Suddenly, important decisions must be made, choices that are in the truest sense, "matters of life and death."

The day-to-day experiences of most people do not prepare them to understand the complexity of this type of decision making environment, much less to function effectively within it. Most patients and their families, like strangers in a foreign land, are bewildered by the traditions, customs, and language of the health care system.

Which one of these doctors is really my doctor?

Why do they have to do surgery just to figure out how to treat me?

What does chemotherapy mean?

Why do I have to be transferred to another hospital to get the treatment I need?

The complexity of the health care system fosters the development of a mystique, particularly when it comes to the treatment of patients with life-threatening illnesses. Patients and families have difficulty penetrating this mystique, and may even come to believe they have no right to do so. As a result, their ability to participate and control what happens to them is extremely limited.

However, the basic thesis of this book is that, given adequate knowledge and information, most people can learn to participate in making choices about their treatment. The assumption that patients and families are incapable of participating in treatment decision making was not supported by our research findings. Rather, their participation was limited largely due to a lack of information and assistance in interpreting what was happening to them. The description provided in this book is directed toward improving consumer knowledge about the health care system, specifically as it effects the treatment of people with life-threatening illnesses. Our description provides both consumers of care and health professionals with a common vocabulary that can be used to communicate about the usual processes and events occurring during treatment decision making. Our goal is to increase the range of options available to patients and families so that choices not to participate in treatment decision making can be made on the basis of personal preference rather than as a result of confusion or lack of information.

Our description is based on actual events that occurred in the lives of real people. The research method we used, participant observation, enabled us to be present as difficult treatment decisions were being made. We could observe what actually happened, and interview key participants to determine their perceptions of events. We also had access to hospital records and other documents where information about treatment decisions, procedures, and protocols is usually recorded. Using all of these sources of information, we developed a comprehensive description of what happens when treatment decisions are made for patients with life-threatening illnesses. The details of our research methods are described in the Appendix.

OVERVIEW

We examine life–death decision making using three different approaches. First, we provide detailed descriptions of each major factor affecting decision making. These factors include: selected elements of health care organization and delivery of services; the availability of medical technology and how it is structured into treatment approaches; who controls decision making and participates in the implementation of treatment; the knowledge and information considered during treatment decision making; the various processes of decision making used; the types of decisions made; and the impact of involvement in life-death decision making on patients, families, and health professionals. The descriptions of each of these factors are illustrated with excerpts from our fieldnotes so that the reader can become a vicarious participant in events.

Next, we provide two case studies to demonstrate how these factors can be used to analyze specific clinical situations with widely divergent characteristics. The cases of baby Bellagio, a premature infant, and Mr. Cathcart, a young man with leukemia, emphasize the dilemmas faced by all participants when making a series of complicated treatment decisions. Finally, we analyze the implications of our description for patients, families, health professionals, and the health care system. We conclude the book by offering a set of practical criteria which any participant in the world of life-death decision making can use in evaluating the quality of health care they have received themselves or offered to others.

CONCLUSION

Some of the case descriptions that follow may disturb the reader, or at least raise issues that require thought and discussion. These situations were similarly stressful and disturbing to the patients and families described in the book who were suddenly hurtled into the world of life-death decision making, and to the caregivers who were trying to help them through these difficult experiences. If the reactions generated by our description are able to spark useful conversation and debate within families, between patients and their caregivers, and among groups of health professionals, then we will have recognized the contribution of all the people who provided data for this study even though they were experiencing some of the most trying times of their lives.

2

THE HEALTH CARE SYSTEM

As we became immersed in the world of life-death decision making, we became increasingly aware of the varied ways the health care system affects how treatment decisions are made for patients with life-threatening illnesses. Indeed, we found this true irrespective of the patient's age, type of disease, or plan of treatment. As a result, an understanding of life-death decision making can only be gained through developing awareness of the structural forces at work within that system. We identified six elements of the health care system which repeatedly played a significant role in the care of life-threatened patients.

The first of these elements, medical rounds, brings together the major participants and emerges as an important vehicle for decision making. Second, while the health care system provides a formal authority structure for decision making, it is the manner in which individual health professionals accept and define their responsibilities that influences the care of life-threatened patients. Third, because the health care system is organized into specialized treatment facilities, seriously ill patients must move along designated pathways, or mobility trajectories, in order to receive appropriate treatment. Fourth, space within specialized facilities is usually restricted, while distances between such facilities can often be great. Fifth, while the health care system is structured to ensure the availability of health personnel, in reality these structures are not always effective. Finally, health care policies give direction to the system, and as a result influence the care of life-threatened patients. Together, these six elements of health care organization create the backdrop against which the drama of life-death decision making unfolds.

5

MEDICAL ROUNDS

In most large treatment centers, decisions for life-threatened patients are made during medical rounds. They can take a variety of forms, such as "chart rounds," "ward rounds," or "X-ray rounds." Attending physicians, residents, interns, and other appropriate members of a medical team meet in specific locales to discuss treatment and care. At the typical ward round, for example, the interns and residents "present" their plans for management of the attending physician's patients for the discussion of all present.

> *The attending doctor arrived on the ward for rounds accompanied by a resident, two interns, and two medical students. The procedure was as follows: the group would go into a patient's room and stand around the bed; the resident would introduce the people who were present and ask the member of the housestaff who admitted the patient to "present" the patient to the group. In one instance, an intern presented all the information on the patient, while in another, the resident asked the patient for the pertinent information and just supplemented it as necessary. Following this, there was a general discussion about the possible causes of the patient's various signs and symptoms as well as the proposed treatment. Before leaving the room, there was some communication with the patient, usually by the attending doctor about the treatment program. On leaving the room, the group would stand in the hall to discuss the patient's condition and treatment plans in more detail.*

The process of "rounding" brings physicians and information together. As a result, rounds are a natural forum for decision making. They are also an educational strategy used by some attending physicians who carefully question interns and residents about their care of patients during the previous 24 hours. In some specialty rounds, consultants who specialize in different fields of medicine collaborate to plan the care of patients requiring complex treatment. While rounds sometimes involve prolonged and intricate discussion of cases, more often they are straightforward presentations of the patient's previous course of treatment and any new plans for the future. The discussions that occur during rounds externalize decision making so that it is accessible to all who attend.

AUTHORITY AND RESPONSIBILITY

The health care system vests control of treatment in the patient's attending physician. This authority is recognized by other health professionals, particularly by medical housestaff, even though they may disagree with the decisions. As one resident observed: "It is the attending physician who makes the decisions, and it is his prerogative to accept or reject advice."

While formal authority clearly resides with the attending physician, not all physicians exercise the responsibilities associated with their role. Indeed, health professionals themselves differ as to what these responsibilities actually entail. When physicians think a colleague is not exercising his responsibility appropriately, they can exert subtle or not so subtle pressure. One physician, who consistently had difficulty with decisions to withdraw treatment, was called in for a "chat" by his service chief whenever such decisions became necessary. The general expectation is that care of the life-threatened patient is a responsibility not to be taken lightly, and any behavior which offends that expectation is a matter of serious concern to physicians and nurses.

MODES OF EXERCISING RESPONSIBILITY

Health professionals tend to accept automatically the responsibilities associated with the care of seriously ill patients. Although responsibilities are delegated to others, the attending physician and his resident are ultimately responsible for ensuring that all assigned activities are carried out. When housestaff (interns and residents) fail in their mandate, they are held accountable.

In caring for life-threatened patients, nurses assume many delegated responsibilities; this is particularly true in specialized units. Adjusting dosages of life-sustaining drugs and weaning patients from respirators are among the activities managed by nurses. These are generally carried out when the criteria for implementing these activities are clear. When difficulties arise, nurses are expected to check with physicians; they know they will be held accountable if they do not. In addition, nurses exercise responsibility by checking orders that they suspect are inaccurate, as well as by channeling and relaying information important to the treatment plan.

Responsibility for care is often transferred from one health professional to another as a patient's changing condition requires different expertise. In other situations, the responsibility for care may not be so smoothly transferred. When a patient is "no longer on active treatment," transfer from a specialized unit can prove difficult if no other medical service wants the patient.

> The attending physician in intensive care asked his residents about transferring the patient to the ward. They were sure no ward resident would be very happy to take the patient. The attending physician suggested that they talk to the chief medical resident and have him assign the patient to a ward. The attending physician commented: "If he makes the decision, then the other people won't be able to do too much about it."

Physicians who understand the formal authority structure will be more successful in achieving their goals than physicians who do not.

DIFFUSION OF RESPONSIBILITY

Although formal authority over care is centralized in the attending physician, in reality responsibility for patient care can become diffused when it is not clear who is exerting control over the therapeutic plan. Diffusion is accentuated by a number of factors: absence of the attending physician; an attending physician's lack of willingness to assume responsibility; or the involvement of a multiplicity of consultants in one patient's care.

> *At rounds, there was discussion about which physician was the patient's attending doctor. When the patient first came in, she was admitted under Dr. Berkeley, a surgeon, who then went on vacation. Dr. Lewis, another surgeon, took over her care. Dr. Lewis consulted the kidney service, which told him that her fluids and electrolytes were not being managed correctly, so they took over her care. At the same time, Dr. Lewis consulted Dr. Stone, a specialist in parenteral nutrition, as well as a urologist because of the patient's bladder problems. During rounds, one of the residents pointed out that he thought Dr. Stone was the attending physician, but another resident disagreed, observing that it was the kidney specialist because his name was on the chart.*

This situation illustrates the difficulties encountered when multiple consultants become involved in the care of a patient. One week after this incident, the consulting urologist called a meeting of all the physicians and housestaff involved in this patient's care, and in a 1½-hour session, they planned the future treatment program. As one resident pointed out, this was the most important contribution anyone could have made to her care.

Diffusion of responsibility has serious implications for health professionals as well as patients and families. When many physicians become involved in the care of one patient, conflicts easily occur as the treatment is planned. As one physician stated: "Not everybody's operating on the same information so one doctor will come along and say that we should do this, and then another will come along and make a different decision because he's operating on different information." Families who hear different opinions about the diagnosis, treatment, and prognosis of their loved one may not know which physician to believe.

Diffusion of responsibility represents a significant problem in the care of life-threatened patients because the resolution of conflicting ideas about what constitutes an effective treatment program may strain interpersonal relationships both among health professionals and between health professionals and their clients. The increasing specialization of physicians makes a major contribution to this problem. As a result, diffusion of responsibility will continue to be a frequent source of frustration for both providers and consumers of care.

MOBILITY TRAJECTORIES

Mobility trajectories are designated pathways along which seriously ill patients must move to receive required health care services. The organization of the health care system into specialized facilities makes such movement necessary. While most people would prefer to be treated in their home or community hospital, the complexity of modern health technology precludes this possibility.

The outcomes of therapy often depend on availability of the appropriate treatment space. For example, a patient might require an isolation room because of low white blood cell counts, or might require emergency surgery. If such space is not available, a mobility trajectory cannot be initiated.

A 70-year-old man was admitted with chronic lymphatic leukemia which was well controlled. He developed a rapidly fulminant but reversible lung problem. Although a lung biopsy was planned, it could not be done because the physicians could not get the patient onto the emergency surgery slate. Treatment was delayed while they were waiting to get the lung biopsy. Unfortunately, when the patient finally went to surgery 48 hours later, he never regained consciousness and died.

When the patient cannot move into the appropriate treatment space, the initiation of therapy can be delayed, with disastrous consequences.

Space is usually not available on short notice, particularly in acute care settings. For example, when patients are found to be seriously ill at an out-patient clinic visit, it can be difficult to find an inpatient bed for them. The need for space often leads to the shifting of patients, creating a chain reaction where the movement of one patient into the system results in the movement of several other patients already within the system.

Because of the continuous problem that health personnel experience over the availability of space, particularly in specialized areas, staff try to keep their units clear of patients who no longer require their services. One nurse who worked in a specialized unit said she had a recurrent fear that some night ten people would land on her ward and she would have no place to put them. Patients who prefer to stay on a particular unit do not always appreciate the staff's insistence on keeping beds open. For example, one man was described as being "afraid to improve too much for fear of being sent home." Similarly, "unloading" of patients from specialized units is not always viewed favorably by the units to which the patients are transferred. As one nurse bluntly stated: "We got an ICU reject today."

At times the appropriate space required by the patient simply does not exist in the system. For example, the need for an intermediate care facility between intensive care units and the general wards was frequently identified by staff. When such places did not exist, staff had to select the "best place" for the patient based on their knowledge of the quality of care on various units.

In many cases, however, patients with life-threatening illnesses follow standard mobility trajectories which have been formulated for their safety. Patients coming into emergency departments with acute chest pain are transferred to coronary care units for cardiac monitoring. All expectant mothers in the northern area are transferred south at 38 weeks gestation because equipment and expertise to resuscitate a baby are not available in remote communities. Patients who have had cardiac arrests and been successfully resuscitated are always transferred to intensive care units. Patients receiving high risk chemotherapy for cancer are admitted to hospitals during their treatment. In this way, certain mobility trajectories are familiar and can be anticipated by health personnel and patients. However, this anticipation results in some trajectories taking on symbolic meaning. For example, one child with cancer refused to move into an isolation room because he thought he would die there. In this case, the child was aware of a standard trajectory; recurrence of disease and resultant low blood counts leading to a move into the isolation room from which some children did not return.

Movement from one space to another frequently requires transitional adjustments. In outlying areas, such adjustments are sometimes elaborate. For example, a two and one-half pound infant born prematurely at a nursing station was transferred after being wrapped in tinfoil and surrounded by hot water bottles. At other times, nurses had to prepare themselves as well as the patient for transport. On a rough flying day, both the patient and the transporting nurse took gravol, an antinauseant medication. Even within the referal hospital, transitional adjustments are required.

> *The nurses brought in the transport incubator to take the baby down for a scan. Virtually every piece of equipment used for the baby's support in the nursery would be taken with him. It took about fifteen minutes to disconnect the infant from his support systems and to get him set up in the transport incubator. Two residents, a nurse and the inhalation therapist accompanied the infant on his trip. The entourage took off from the nursery, wheeling the incubator with all its attachments as well as portable oxygen and suction equipment. All the way the nurse listened to the baby's heart with the stethoscope while a resident ventilated the infant.*

If transitional adjustments are inappropriate, the consequences for the life-threatened patient can be drastic. In one instance, a high risk baby was transferred by ambulance from an outlying area to the referal hospital without an incubator and unattended by a physician or nurse. The baby stopped breathing several times en route, and subsequently died of a brain hemorrhage.

Even when death is the anticipated outcome, failure to make appropriate transitional adjustments can have unpleasant outcomes. In one instance, a patient with cancer died at home after a long illness. When he was subsequently taken to the hospital to be pronounced dead, health personnel attempted to resuscitate him. To avoid such inappropriate treatment when a terminally ill patient has chosen to die at home, some community health nurses ask the attending physician to come to the home to "pronounce" the patient after death has occurred.

The initiation of a mobility trajectory often forces the separation of the patient from his family. Family members who are unable to accompany their loved one to the hospital are particularly vulnerable to feelings of helplessness.

It was a bumpy ride down to the airstrip for the two patients who were being flown out. The plane was waiting when we got there, and the two stretchers were loaded quite easily onto the plane. The mother of the young girl with suspected appendicitis went into the plane to say goodbye. The nurse asked the wife of the man with lower limb paralysis whether she also wanted to say goodbye before the plane left. This woman became very upset, pulled away from the nurse, and ran over to the edge of the airstrip where she stood with her back to us, obviously crying. Then they closed the doors and the plane took off into the bright summer sky. The woman watched the plane as it disappeared with the tears still streaming down her face. As we all watched the plane finally disappear over the forest, I sensed the uncertainty that the others were feeling. We were all wondering what was going to happen to those two sick people, and whether we would ever see them again.

LIMITED SPACE AND EXTENDED DISTANCE

In many specialized treatment facilities, the geographical area within which care must be delivered is extremely small. Restricted space has some unpleasant consequences for life-threatened patients. In open units, patients sometimes observe the deaths of other patients, although staff usually try to shield them from observing active treatment interventions such as resuscitation. On the other hand, restricted geographic space has some definite advantages. In the open areas of specialized units where all patients can be easily seen, impending trouble can be quickly observed and intervention promptly initiated. Similarly, discussions about patient care are readily accessible to anyone present, and there is ample opportunity for clarification of treatment decisions.

The distance between specialized facilities for care of life-threatened patients affects the quality of health services. If the various treatment areas are close to each other, such as on the labor and delivery floor, patients who experience a sudden crisis can be transported within seconds to life-saving equipment and services. On the other hand, when the distance is great, even very ill patients may have to travel to receive specialized treatments. Extended distance requires that treatment be adapted to rapidly changing circumstances, with complex care being administered in airplanes and ambulances. Extended distance also produces increased risk and discomfort for patients.

AVAILABILITY OF HEALTH PERSONNEL

Within the health care system, organizational structures have been developed to ensure that the health personnel required for care of seriously ill patients are available. For example, "on call" systems provide housestaff with backup from more experienced physicians. Nursing schedules are designed to provide sufficient nursing personnel on a 24-hour basis.

At times, however, appropriate personnel are not available, and this lack of availability can have serious consequences. Weekends and holidays present particular problems.

> *The resident explained to me that he had a problem. Intensive care wants to transfer a patient down to the ward. However, with the long weekend starting this evening, the head nurse on the ward won't take the patient because they want his I.P.P.B. (breathing treatment) done every half hour and she doesn't have enough staff. The resident said that the intensive care people just don't understand that the ward nurses can't do treatments that often on the weekend. He laughed and added: "I might be there over the weekend doing the I.P.P.B. myself."*

Shortages of personnel have a direct effect on the quality of health care received by the seriously ill patient. For example, physicians are usually reluctant to make major changes in treatment while the patient's attending physician is away. However, if such a decision is required, another staffperson may be asked to consult.

> *Dr. Mead explained that during the summer he frequently receives calls from other hospitals regarding decisions to remove treatment. The reason for this is that the attending doctors are on vacation, and the doctors taking their places don't know the patients very well. Therefore, they call him to get a second opinion.*

Problems in availability of personnel leads to a variety of adjustments in care delivery. For example, if physicians are not readily available, nurses must assume more responsibility for treatment decisions. If staff perceive that a "competent" specialist is not available to treat a patient, they may design treatment to keep a patient alive until another specialist can be consulted. When the attending physician is temporarily absent, residents frequently have to make difficult decisions about tests or treatment.

While organizational frameworks have been developed to ensure availability of health personnel, in practice they do not always function effectively, especially on nights, weekends, and during vacations. Although various adjustments may be made to safeguard the care of patients, these adjustments are not always adequate to protect patients from the untoward consequences of staffing problems.

HEALTH CARE POLICIES

Health care policies are the rules and regulations that direct the function of the system. The process of treatment for life-threatened patients is affected by many of these policies. For example, one important institutional policy requires that all patients who experience a cardiac arrest be resuscitated. Other policies restrict the use of specialized equipment to specific hospital units. Policy manuals on some specialized units outline the "privileges" accorded attending physicians. Policies governing admission to specialized units attempt to restrict admissions only to those patients who can benefit from the services of that unit. In general, health care policies function to protect the rights and well being of patients.

However, there are obvious instances when institutional policies conflict with reality. For example, when a patient is dying and all aggressive treatment has been discontinued, the "resuscitate all" policy does not make much sense. For that reason, decisions are made not to resuscitate some patients in spite of the institutional policy. Similarly, restrictions on the use of specialized equipment are sometimes not realistic, and negotiations with administration are required to have policies waived in special cases. In other instances, admission policies are ignored when a patient is in exceptional circumstances.

> *Dr. Archibald said that this lady was an exceptional admission. Normally, they reject emergency admissions of unknown origin, but they had accepted this patient and would just have to take the policy consequences. He said there was a great deal of sympathy for the patient because she had a terrible, smelly wound and was in a lot of pain. They didn't want to send her elsewhere because it would mean another ambulance ride.*

Policies tend to be formulated to deal with the "usual" case. When policies conflict with the patient's best interest, health professionals try to circumvent them.

CONCLUSION

While health professionals are generally familiar with various aspects of health care organization, the ones we have described are those that have the greatest impact on life–death decision making. These aspects of health care organization will be less familiar to patients and families. Both providers and consumers of care need to recognize the pervasive influence these six components have on how treatment decisions are actually made for patients with life-threatening illnesses.

The life-threatened patient and his family need to understand how the treatment system functions if they are to participate in life–death decision making. Generally, patients and families are unaware of these aspects, and as a result, are powerless to manipulate the system to their advantage. The health care system is the social reality within which health professionals operate, and it is their knowledge of that system that gives them power. The more knowledge patients and families acquire about the health care system, the better they will be able to communicate with health professionals and influence the process of treatment planning.

Health professionals need to recognize that difficulties in life–death decision making may be related to structures and processes of the health care system. In their day-to-day practice, physicians in particular get caught up in the details of individual cases. As a result, they may fail to recognize the influence that the system is exerting on their processes of decision making. The quality of life–death decision making cannot be adequately assessed without considering the context within which it occurs.

As our description continues, the reader will become increasingly aware of the influence of health care organization on the processes of life–death decision making.

3

TECHNOLOGY AND TREATMENT

While the care of every life-threatened patient is influenced by the health care system, specific treatment is highly dependent on the availability of medical technology. Rapid developments in medical science have led to the widespread use of drugs, equipment, and procedures that were unknown or at least highly experimental even 25 years ago. Traditionally, improvements in medicine were aimed at cure of acute diseases. Today, many techniques have been developed to control a disease state or its effects while not producing a cure. The extent to which new medical techniques are available to the public has a significant influence on therapeutic decision making.

When appropriate health technology is available, the type of care received by a patient depends on how it is structured into treatment plans. Such plans usually include a series of "tries" to see what treatment approach will work. This is necessary because a treatment approach that proves to be successful for one patient is not necessarily equally effective for another patient. Generally, treatment plans have either a curative or a palliative intent. A curative trial is a treatment plan aimed at eradicating disease or restoring function; its intent is to preserve life. On the other hand, the goal of a palliative trial or treatment plan is to provide physical, psychological, and social comfort in the face of progressive disease, recognizing that death may be inevitable.

AVAILABILITY OF TECHNOLOGY

The range of medical procedures, equipment, and drugs available to practitioners and patients has expanded rapidly over the past few decades. Experienced health personnel can see the changes that have occurred during their years of practice. For example, one chemotherapy nurse recalled that when she started in the specialty there were only two or three drugs available for cancer treatment, whereas now there are dozens. Patients also recognize the effect of improvements in technology on their treatment. One man who was offered coronary bypass surgery stated that he was really happy his problem had not occurred 10 years ago when this surgical procedure was not available.

The advent of new technology is an ongoing process that affects the design of treatment. For example, the acquisition of computerized axial tomography in Manitoba was welcomed by practitioners because it simplified the diagnosis of serious disorders such as intracranial lesions. Health personnel quickly adjust their therapeutic trials to include the use of new technology which they view as improving care of the seriously ill patient.

LIMITATIONS ON THE AVAILABILITY OF TECHNOLOGY

Health personnel are sometimes limited in the drugs or treatments they can use as diagnostic or treatment options. A new drug, for example, may be difficult to obtain because of its limited supply and the "red tape" required to get approval for its use. At times, pragmatic considerations influence availability.

During Friday's rounds there was discussion about a patient with a suspected abdominal abscess. The resident wanted a gallium scan of her abdomen, but the gallium would not be available until Monday. He wanted an echogram instead, but the doctor in charge of that test was away until Monday. Being unable to get these tests, he went ahead with liver, lung, and spleen scans.

Another practical consideration is efficient equipment maintenance. If a piece of equipment breaks down and is not repaired quickly, it may not be available when needed.

The availability of specific technology may also be limited by social, medical, or legal acceptability. For example, a patient with an indwelling urinary catheter may not be able to return home if the family finds the catheter socially unacceptable. Physicians prefer medically proven treatments over newer treatments that have uncertain or questionable benefits; the latter may also be legally unacceptable.

Heavy demand on specialized equipment may be a limiting factor. For example, on the labor floor the number of women requiring fetal monitoring may exceed the number of monitors available.

The nurse decided on a way to allocate the monitors because all the patients were high risk. Theoretically, all should have been monitored but there were only three monitors available. So, she decided that the patient with the elevated temperature and fetal heart rate of 168 should be monitored to get a baseline reading. Then she would move that monitor to the newly admitted patient with premature ruptured membranes. By logically priorizing each woman's need, she was able to "make do."

In remote areas, limitations on the availability of technology are particularly apparent. For example, patients who require even simple blood tests to monitor acute conditions are often flown out for such testing procedures. In isolated settlements, the shortwave radio and airplane are important elements of medical technology.

The nurses described a man with a head injury: he had a large hematoma and was breathing irregularly. A plane was about to leave the settlement so they tried to radio the pilot to wait for this patient to come to the airstrip. But they couldn't reach him and he took off moments before the nurses reached the airstrip with the patient. The nurses then had to wait with the patient, who periodically stopped breathing, for 2½ hours before a chartered plane arrived.

Often sophisticated technology is accessible only through physicians who are specially trained in its use, and its availability is at the discretion of the specialist. For example, a specialist may withhold the service if it looks like a particular technique will not benefit the patient. The patient or attending physician may then have to negotiate with the specialist if they wish the technique made available.

One case discussed at mortality rounds was that of an 18-year-old woman with diabetes complicated by congestive heart failure. About six hours before her death a decision had been made to stop aggressive treatment. The intensive care physicians had asked the renal service to initiate dialysis; but this was refused. The resident said they then withdrew treatment because there were no other options left.

The nature of the procedure, equipment, or drug itself can limit its availability. Some treatments, such as chemotherapy and radiotherapy, have intrinsic limitations on their use. Physicians become frustrated when they have "used up" all possible effective drugs or have already given the patient as much radiation as they can. Patients also recognize that as their disease progresses, treatment options become increasingly limited. For example, one woman with cancer recognized that she could not get any more radiation and that the only treatment option left to her was chemotherapy. For other patients, such as infants with brain hemorrhages or viral meningitis, there is no effective treatment at all.

Cost may limit the availability of technology in specific circumstances. The high cost of a procedure sometimes leads to careful consideration as to whether or not it should be used. For example, if the information gained from an expensive test will not influence treatment plans, health personnel may be asked to justify its need.

Because every health professional encounters situations when access to technology is limited, a number of strategies have evolved to overcome this difficulty. Sometimes physicians or nurses convince their colleagues that a situation is an emergency in order to get access to technology that has a limited availability. At the institutional level, the use of backup systems (such as extra resuscitation carts) ensures that the equipment is available even if the first system breaks down. Governmental strategies such as legalization of certain drugs and the introduction of pre-paid medical insurance programs are viewed by both health personnel and consumers as improving the availability of health care. Whether these strategies are effective or not, participants in life–death decision making generally expect that no one will limit access when it is genuinely needed for the care of the seriously ill patient.

THE CURATIVE TRIAL

Planning therapy for the life-threatened person involves outlining or structuring health technology into treatment trials. Cure, or the irradication of disease, is the usual intent of these trials. Curative trials can be straightforward, such as the use of an antibiotic to cure an infection; or very complex, as when a patient has two or more illnesses, each of which has several treatment alternatives.

A 32-year-old woman had Stage II breast cancer which was treated by mastectomy. She also had kidney problems and had just recently recovered from TB. The physician suggested the following plan for her cancer: (1) if the disease had spread to her liver then she should have surgery to remove her ovaries so that the development of the tumor would not be fostered by hormones secreted from the ovaries; (2) if her cancer regressed after this surgery, she should be put on chemotherapy to prevent recurrence of the disease; (3) in any case the patient should go on drugs to prevent a flare-up of her TB; (4) if the liver test showed no spread of the cancer, she should just go on the antituberculosis drugs and chemotherapy; and (5) in view of the cell type of her cancer and if no spread of the disease was discovered, she should have the other breast removed because of the very high chance of it becoming cancerous as well. The physician added that he would consult the patient's kidney specialist and her tuberculosis doctor because he would need their cooperation in planning her treatment.

Defining the adequate time span for a curative trial can also present difficulties.

A young man with acute leukemia has been in remission since his diagnosis two years ago, and continues to do well. Dr. Hastings, his attending physician, was asked when he would take this patient off treatment: "I really don't know. Right now I'm happy with the response I've got." He added that a similar patient had relapsed after he lengthened the intervals between treatments, and that another doctor's patient had relapsed after being off treatment for 1½ years.

Often technology has to be removed to determine whether or not a trial has been successful. For example, during cardiopulmonary resuscitation, an endotracheal tube is usually inserted to facilitate artificial ventilation. Eventually, this tube is removed to see if the patient can breathe without it. In other instances, drugs are removed to determine the status of an underlying condition. For example, health personnel treating an infant for seizures may discontinue the antiseizure drug to see if the problem has been resolved. In other situations, the removal of technology is accomplished gradually, such as when a patient is weaned from a respirator. If a physician perceives the length of a previous trial as inadequate, a repeat may be ordered. In this sense, arriving at the appropriate duration of a trial is important because an alternative treatment plan, from which the patient might benefit, can be delayed while a trial is being repeated.

In trials which require combining several treatment modalities, the sequencing of these modalities is often critical to the success or failure of the trial. For example, in the treatment of patients with certain cancers, the sequencing of radiotherapy and surgery is important.

A patient with cancer of the larynx was receiving radiotherapy, but at examination the radiotherapist found no change in tumor size. The radiotherapist and the surgeon agreed that the radiation was not working. The surgeon said radiation usually decreases the size of these tumors, but added that in this case he thought the radiation was a "forlorn hope." The radiotherapist agreed, and said he would stop the treatments so the patient would be ready for surgery in a week.

One treatment modality may influence the next in the sequence, rendering it more or less effective. For example, one surgeon stopped an antibiotic for a patient he suspected of having an abdominal abscess so the abscess would be more prominent and therefore easier to find at surgery. Defining the sequence of treatments within a curative trial is a crucial component in planning care for the seriously ill patient.

THE STANDARD PREPLANNED TRIAL

The standard preplanned trial is a type of curative trial. Frequently referred to as a "treatment protocol," this approach has been described and widely accepted by health professionals. A variety of treatment protocols exist for patients with specific diseases: protocols for patients with low white blood cell counts, with lead intoxication, with severe high blood pressure during pregnancy, and with hepatic coma. Patients receiving certain treatments such as parenteral nutrition, are also placed on protocols.

The group of patients who are most consistently entered into planned treatment protocols are those with cancer. Specific protocols are available for patients with cancer of various sites (breast, lung, etc.), of various cell types (sarcomas, epidermoid cancers, etc.), and of various stages (degrees of the cancer in the body). If a treatment protocol exists for a patient with a particular type and stage of cancer, the patient receives the sequence of therapy specified in the description of the protocol. This description usually includes diagrams of the sequencing of treatments within the trial at specific daily, weekly or monthly intervals.

The general aim of treatment protocols is to ensure that patients are given the greatest possibility of cure for their diseases; or, if that is not possible, to ensure prolonged survival. If the patient agrees to be part of an "experimental" protocol, that is, one designed to establish the relative effectiveness of various treatments for a given disease, the patient will be "randomized" to determine which of the treatment sequences described in the protocol will be followed. Randomization means that the sequence of therapy the patient actually receives is determined by chance.

At times, however, the nature of the patient's disease is such that it is difficult to find the appropriate treatment protocol.

A woman with Stage III cancer of the breast was described at rounds. The surgeon had been unable to excise all the tumor because it was wrapped around a group of blood vessels. The radiotherapist and chemotherapist looked at the treatment protocols for patients with breast cancer, and found there was none to fit this patient. They were concerned that the chemotherapy in the existing protocols would not be strong enough for their patient who still had some tumor left.

In other cases, treatment protocols are modified if patients develop severe side effects of treatment such as very low blood counts, or complications such as bleeding or infection.

THE NEWLY CREATED TRIAL

Another type of curative trial is the "newly created" trial. This arises when new technology, information, knowledge or skill are incorporated into preexisting treatment approaches or when an entirely new approach to treatment is formulated. A newly created trial usually comes into being when existing treatment approaches are viewed as inadequate, or when all existing approaches have been exhausted.

> *The resident explained that Mrs. Hudd had thrombocytopenia (low platelets, which are required for blood clotting). Although she had this illness for a long time, it became progressively severe over the past two years and now threatened her life. He said they had exhausted all the known ways of treating her without any success. Finally they tried giving her platelets prepared by a new technique in their lab, but this treatment approach also failed.*

Although new treatment approaches are unsuccessful more often than not, the newly created trial which proves effective for one or more patients may eventually be standardized into a treatment protocol. In no small measure, creation of a new trial depends on the ingenuity of the practitioner, and is a source of pride if it is successful.

THE ROUTINE TRIAL

The routine trial is a standardized treatment automatically initiated in response to a particular event or chain of events. The most frequent example of a routine curative trial is cardiopulmonary resuscitation. When a person suffers cardiopulmonary collapse in hospital, most patients are resuscitated. Staff roles in initiating this routine trial are clearly defined, and if they fail to play their roles adequately they are usually held accountable.

INDIVIDUALLY PLANNED TRIAL

The individually planned trial takes into account not only accepted treatment modalities but the values, needs and lifestyles of the patient and his family. Examples of individually planned curative trials are most frequently observed in outpatient clinics, but also occur in high technology environments such as intensive care units. For example, in one such unit the method of weaning a patient from the respirator was specially designed to minimize his anxiety.

There are many examples to illustrate how outpatient treatment is designed around the lifestyles of patients. Therapy may be scheduled early in the morning for patients concerned about being able to get to work on time. Treatment options offered to patients may be modified because of job requirements. For example, one man with cancer of the throat was offered radiation rather than radical surgery because he was a lecturer and needed a strong voice. Nurses may be sent to homes to draw blood samples from seriously ill patients when it is clear that travel will only add to discomfort. If possible, rural patients are given oral drugs rather than intravenous ones in order to reduce their travel requirements. Psychological factors are also important in planning trials. For example, if a patient is under considerable psychological stress, drug dosages may be altered to prevent additional physical distress from the side effects of the treatment. Additionally, health professionals view planning treatment around holidays, particularly Christmas, as an extremely important obligation.

> *The nurse was looking through her appointment book, and pointed out the names of patients who required treatments around Christmas. She said they try to avoid treatments on Christmas or New Year's, and instead schedule them a few days earlier or a few days later. She pointed to the name of one patient in the book, a young woman with breast cancer who has two children, saying, "It's really important for her not to be sick at Christmas." This woman was always nauseated after her treatment, so the nurse planned to ask the physician if her treatment might be put off until after the holidays.*

However, issues of sensitivity aside, there are other factors which determine whether or not treatment should be altered in response to a special request.

> *In dictating his note on a young man with leukemia, Dr. Curry stated: "The patient asked to have chemotherapy deferred for one week and we will comply with this request." After clinic, Dr. Curry explained this patient's request and how he decided to grant it. He said there were three factors: (1) how well the treatment was controlling the disease; (2) the degree of flexibility of treatment schedules in the protocol; and (3) the nature of the patient's request. In the case of this young man there was no problem granting his request because there was a fair degree of flexibility in his treatment schedules. He contrasted this situation with that of a young woman with trophoblastic cancer. She had wanted her treatment postponed until after a wedding she wanted to attend. Dr. Curry said, "In her disease the treatment schedules are rigidly defined, so I can't grant her request." Although she had to take her treatment as scheduled before the wedding, Dr. Curry arranged for her to see a physician in the city where the wedding was held just in case there were problems arising from the treatment.*

At times, when the patient's disease progresses so rapidly that health professionals must ignore lifestyle factors in planning treatment, they feel badly. For example, when aggressive testing and treatment was planned for a patient over the Christmas holidays, one physician glumly remarked, "What a Christmas present."

THE PALLIATIVE TRIAL

When cure or restoration of function is not possible, palliative or comfort-oriented trials may be initiated. While comfort care occurs more frequently in patients near the end of their lives, curative therapy may also be altered in anticipation of the later need for palliative care. For example, some patients with cancer receive home visits from nurses when progression of their disease is anticipated. In this way, a relationship is established between the family and home care service, so that timing the onset of palliative treatment can be accurately determined. In such situations, the transition from aggressive treatment to comfort care occurs smoothly, as health personnel, patient and family realize that the disease is irreversible and can no longer be controlled.

However, in many cases this transition does not occur, and curative therapy continues until the time of death.

> *A 73-year-old man with acute leukemia was treated with chemotherapy and subsequently developed infections in his bladder, lung, and knee. He also developed heart failure. The patient stated that he wanted to die, but the unit physicians continued active treatment, consulting intensive care and placing the patient on the granulocytopenic (low white blood cell) protocol. The nurses were told to give the patient's heart drug intravenously if he could not take it orally. The patient died later that day.*

Characteristics of the illness itself can influence whether or not the transition to palliative care occurs. If the patient has a sudden, acute illness, treatment often remains curative in intent even though at some point the prognosis becomes "hopeless." In contrast, gradual deterioration sometimes enables health personnel and the family to make the transition to palliative care.

Palliative treatment modalities may easily be mistaken for those with a curative intent. For example, cancer chemotherapy and radiotherapy may be used with either a palliative or a curative intent. Health personnel, patients, and families are prone to identify both chemotherapy and radiotherapy as having only a curative function, while in fact they are often used to control pain and alleviate other symptoms.

THE STANDARD PREPLANNED PALLIATIVE TRIAL

An important preplanned trial for patients with chronic pain due to cancer uses oral narcotics on a regular rather than PRN (as the patient needs it) basis. On one unit, patients who were admitted on intramuscular morphine were always switched to oral morphine for pain control.

> *Dr. Walters said there were reasons why he preferred to switch patients from parenteral to oral administration. He said he was influenced one morning when a night nurse told him she had given 40 injections that night. He said patients receiving so many injections tend to get sore,*

infected injection sites and that makes them more uncomfortable.
He added that taking the drug orally was "more elegant" and decreased
the patient's sense of dependency on the staff.

Nurses on this unit were aware of the use of the pain control protocol
as a method of preventing pain by giving analgesics regularly, and they taught
this approach to patients and families.

INDIVIDUALLY PLANNED PALLIATIVE TRIALS

Understandably, most comfort oriented trials are individually planned for
patients. Because of the high stress associated with some symptoms such as pain,
a variety of approaches are tried to bring it under control.

Dr. Lake described a female patient who had shortness of breath,
problems moving, and pain. He noted they managed to control the
first two, and were bringing the pain under control, but the pain
treatment made her drowsy. He suggested to the patient that radio-
therapy might provide pain relief without drowsiness, but she resisted
because the last time she had radiotherapy it made her quite sick.

Planning for holidays is also important in comfort-oriented care. For
example, one patient with very low hemoglobin was given blood transfusions
so she would not faint during Christmas festivities. Even small discomforts,
such as poorly fitting dentures, can become a focus for individually planned
care.

One patient who was dying was upset about the fact that her dentures
were not fitting, so a dentist was called. He put in a temporary liner and
was going to return later to finish the job correctly. The dentist
explained that the lady really wanted new dentures, but this is unreal-
istic in terms of her prognosis.

Planning for the comfort of individual patients requires the cooperation
of a wide variety of health personnel.

CONCLUSION

While a variety of health care technology is available, how it becomes structured
into trials is a crucial element in life–death decision making. In order to understand the nature of their treatment, patients and families need to be aware of
the intent of the trial. In addition, they need to be aware that even standardized
treatment approaches can be modified in recognition of the patient's concerns

and lifestyle. Patients and families must become active participants in the treatment process for such modifications to occur.

Practitioners are probably justified in expecting access to whatever technology they require. At the same time, once the technology is available, it will be used whenever appropriate. The structuring of technology into standardized treatment protocols creates pressures to implement the technology, and fosters a self-perpetuating system of intervention-oriented care. Current institutional and governmental restraints in the acquisition and allocation of technology may provide some limits on the extent to which this ethos can be pursued in the future.

The technological emphasis in modern health care explains why we observed so few comfort-oriented trials outside the palliative care unit. The orientation of most health professionals remains profoundly curative. In terms of its potential impact on patient comfort and dignity, this emphasis on the curative, at the expense of the palliative aspects of patient care, needs to be reevaluated.

4

CONTROL AND PARTICIPATION

Many participants in life–death decisions attempt to exercise control over the design of therapy. We will describe four patterns of control: provider-controlled, patient-controlled, family-controlled, and jointly-controlled decision making. Whoever has control determines the selection of treatment options, and the structure and intent of the trial. The "controller" of the trial inevitably participates in some way in its implementation. However, participation does not necessarily imply control.

In most situations, medical staff exercise final control over the design of treatment. Nurses rarely control decision making for the seriously ill, except when they occupy administrative positions or are the only health personnel available. Patients and families can exercise control over treatment plans, but are often unable to do so for a variety of reasons. While some patients express their wishes with respect to the design of treatment, only the most insistent are successful if their plan differs from that of health personnel.

PROVIDER–CONTROLLED DECISION MAKING

In provider-controlled decision making, health personnel exercise final control over the design of treatment. While some providers of care use this approach to decision making only when the patient and family are unable or unwilling to participate, others practice the approach regularly and view it as appropriate.

The physician said it was not appropriate for the family to be involved in the decision to treat this elderly man with extensive pelvic cancer.

27

He said they wouldn't have the information that would enable them to make a decision about radical surgery or dialysis. But he added: "Maybe they could make a suggestion on an emotional basis, to keep on treating or to stop treatment."

One way of implementing provider-controlled decision making is for the physician to present a decision as the "best choice" to the patient and family without discussing other alternatives. Another strategy is to present the decision, and then to ask the patient or family if they disagree. This was the approach used in decisions to stop treatment in one intensive care area.

Dr. Street said they generally make the decision, then communicate it to the family and ask whether or not they agree. Whenever he has asked the family to decide, they usually come back to him and ask him to make the decision. Families have told him they don't have the information or background to make that kind of decision. He said that he and one of his colleagues believe the same approach should be used with the patient who is alert. In other words, you should inform the patient of the treatment plan and its consequences. Dr. Street said that some patients will say, "Okay, go ahead;" others won't say anything; and still others will say, "No, I'd like you to try something else." He was serious as he said this, pausing to reflect for a few minutes in silence before describing by way of example the patient who died yesterday after they discontinued treatment. Apparently, the surgeon had just wanted to give the patient some morphine so he would go to sleep and then die after treatment was stopped. However, Dr. Street disagreed, and instead explained the decision to the patient.

In other situations, patients and families do not even have veto power over ongoing treatment decisions. For example, in one intensive care area, the fact that decisions to stop treatment were being made by staff was not explicitly communicated to family members. Thus, some seriously ill patients were disconnected from life support systems without family members being told of the decision. Health professionals justified this as appropriate because it "protects" the family.

The head nurse said that it was a medical decision based on medical knowledge, and the family could not even begin to comprehend what was going on. She said, "Why give them that guilt to live with?" She added that some young doctors tried to get family members involved in the decision making in the past, but because of their bad experiences she doubted whether they would try again.

Emotional protection of the family members from the guilt of decision making is the usual justification given by health personnel for making treatment decisions on behalf of patients and families. This motivation is most intense when the life of a child is at stake.

Providers are able to exercise this high degree of control for a variety of reasons. In many instances, patients and families simply do not want to participate and trust health personnel completely with treatment decisions.

A young woman with Hodgkin's disease said she had never participated in the decisions about her treatment: because she had implicit trust in her physician, she said she accepted the decisions that were made for her.

Physicians who carefully explain treatment options and ask the patient to participate are often told, "That's up to you, doctor." These patients do not expect to participate in decision making, and choose not to even if the opportunity presents itself. Other patients perceive that they simply do not have much choice because of the seriousness of their illness.

PATIENT–CONTROLLED DECISION MAKING

Some life-threatened patients are successful in controlling the design of their treatment. Withholding consent is one way to achieve control. For example, one elderly woman steadfastly refused to have surgery for her bowel obstruction, in spite of the fact that numerous physicians, family members, and her priest appealed to her in attempts to change her mind. In this case, the patient was judged to be mentally alert and therefore competent to withhold her consent. Other patients are also effective in gaining control over treatment through sheer stubbornness.

A 55-year-old man with chest pain and tingling in his arms, kept going to his doctor who repeatedly said his cardiogram was fine and told him to keep taking nitros. Then the man's bad pain brought him to emergency, only to be sent home because they couldn't find anything on the cardiogram. A day later the pain was worse and the patient returned to emergency. Again, they wanted to send him home. This time the patient said he was not going anywhere until he saw a cardiologist. The cardiologist who finally looked at the cardiogram sent the man to intensive care. Apparently, the pattern in his cardiogram was unusually difficult to read. In later discussing this incident, the patient emphasized that he would have been discharged and might have died if he had not insisted on seeing the cardiologist.

A variety of creative strategies are used by patients to gain control. One young woman, upset about her chemotherapy treatment for Hodgkin's disease, missed her clinic appointment and instead wrote her physician a letter stating her viewpoint. He then invited her to return to the clinic to discuss her ideas, stating in his letter, "I do understand your feelings and feel at least partly responsible that we did not talk about them during one of your clinic visits." After their discussion, the treatment plan was changed to the one proposed in the patient's letter. During an interview, this young woman expressed her views on planning treatment.

> *She said she was the kind of person who really wanted to know what was going to happen and when it was going to happen. She thought this was particularly important for young people. She added that she had young children to care for and it was important to her to be able to fulfill her responsibilities as a mother. That was why she wanted to try going without the treatment she had been on for eight months.*

Patients are more likely to gain control over treatment design if they are given the opportunity to participate in decision making. For example, life-threatened patients who might benefit from elective surgery are given ample opportunity to give or withhold consent. One cardiologist approached patients to see if they would consent to surgery before even starting the complicated pre-operative tests. Other physicians clearly outline the various treatment approaches that could be pursued, and leave the final decision to the patient. However, in most instances, physicians indicate the choice that they believe to be best. While many patients are content to have health professionals make treatment decisions on their behalf, some are not and attempt to gain control over the decision making process.

FAMILY–CONTROLLED DECISION MAKING

Families can exert control over the design of treatment for the seriously ill patient. Usually, such control is exercised by refusing consent. For example, one family withheld consent for insertion of a pacemaker in their elderly father who had undergone aggressive treatment over several weeks. Parents of children with congenital abnormalities sometimes withhold consent for life-saving surgery. Health personnel recognize that families have this control, and in some situations hope they will exercise it.

> *The resident said that a very sick 83-year-old man was having problems with his bowels and his tube feedings. He remarked, "I'm just waiting for something to happen. Then I'll go to the family for permission to insert some tube or monitoring line. When they say no, well. . ." and he shrugged his shoulders and smiled.*

In other cases, families influence health personnel to respect the previously stated wishes of the patient.

The patient had been in intensive care with a chest problem two years previously. After that experience, he told his children that he never wanted to go on a respirator again. The family thought that if he were conscious, their father would want the treatment stopped. The attending physician concurred with the family's request to stop aggressive treatment.

JOINTLY-CONTROLLED DECISION MAKING

Control over the treatment design may also be shared. In contrast to provider-controlled decision making, the exercise of joint control assumes that patients and families are capable of participating in life-death decision making without sustaining undue psychological damage.

Dr. Erikson described baby Gregg with the words: "Much poorer. The baby is bleeding into his brain and seizuring. Even if he lives, he'll be severely brain damaged." He went on to say the parents were coming in shortly. Then, he became reflective and said, "If this were mine to decide, I'd take the baby off the respirator. I'm going to talk to the parents about that." Later the parents came into the nursery after their meeting with the physician. They asked the nurse if they could hold their baby. The nurse told them if they held the baby, the baby would have to come off the respirator, and he would die. The parents said that was alright with them. The nurse took the baby off the respirator. He died in his mother's arms.

STRATEGIES AND TACTICS

A number of strategies and tactics are used by participants in life-death decision making to help themselves or others gain control over the design of treatment. Health professionals have a number of formal processes for achieving such control. One is the use of blanket consent forms. For example, infants and children transported from northern communities were frequently sent with a consent to treatment already signed. One transfer sheet designed to accompany ill newborns to a referal center included a request to "have parents sign attached consent form." Health staff could then make decisions about the care of the infant without necessarily consulting the parents. One father was surprised, when he went to a regional hospital to visit his baby, to find that the baby had been transferred to a teaching hospital more than 500 miles away without his knowledge.

In addition, health personnel use a variety of informal tactics to gain control.

At rounds they discussed a patient who had been in a car accident and was critically injured. She had been "hidden," as one of the residents put it, in a corner of the intensive care area by her surgeon, who wanted to treat the patient's deteriorating respiratory status conservatively, without having to consult any of his colleagues. However, an attending respirologist found this patient while walking around the unit, and subsequently convinced the surgeon to let him consult on the case.

In this case, the surgeon's tactic was not successful. In others, physicians enlist the assistance of colleagues to convince families to follow their treatment recommendations. For example, one community doctor did not want to treat a patient with cancer, but the family kept pushing him to order chemotherapy. The physician consulted a cancer specialist, and asked him to write a letter expressing his opinion so it could be shown to the family.

Nurses also use a variety of tactics to gain control over treatment. In the following example, one physician refused to leave adequate orders for pain control on his terminally ill patients, but the nurses devised a way to administer the drugs anyway.

This doctor does not believe in giving his dying patients regular narcotics and writes them as a PRN (only as necessary) order. However, the nurses tend to give them at regular intervals. They do this by writing out a medication ticket that says "PRN, check every four hours." Then, if they know the patient needs the medication every four hours, the nurses just prepare the medication, and take it in to the patient. As the nurses said, "After all, a PRN order means it's a matter of judgement whether or not the patient needs the medication."

In this case, the nurses believed that these patients "needed" the narcotics regularly, and so they gave them regularly. In other situations, nurses are quick to act on a physician's order before he can change his mind.

The nurse explained to the resident why she thought the infant's nasogastric tube could be removed. He told her to go ahead and remove it. The nurse said later that she removed the tube as quickly as she could in case he changed his mind. Sure enough, the resident came back two minutes later and said, "Maybe we had better just clamp the tube for a couple of hours and see how she does." The nurse had replied, "Sorry, too late, it's already out."

Another tactic used by nurses is to ignore treatment orders with which they do not agree. For example, one nurse who was asked by a physician to remove the pink tag (symbol for no resuscitation) from a patient's nursing record simply failed to do so. She then went off duty for several days without informing other nurses of the physician's request.

Children are particularly creative in the tactics they use to get some control over their treatment. They bargain with staff members: "I will do X if you will (or will not) do Y." They threaten not to eat unless the adults comply with their wishes. Children also take matters into their own hands when the adults around them prove ineffective.

A boy with severe congenital heart disease came to the nursing station for treatment. He and a nurse tried to fly out on one of the planes, but there was only one seat, so they couldn't go. When the next plane came in, they found that the child was missing. Apparently, he had taken his transfer papers, walked back to the airfield, and left on the first plane. When the plane landed in the city, he went to the hospital with his papers in his hand. They later found out he had taken this initiative because of his own concern for his health and his lack of faith in the adults around him to act effectively.

Children tended to be less inhibited than adults in challenging the system, and as a result they succeeded in getting their own way in a surprising number of cases.

PARTICIPATION IN THE IMPLEMENTATION OF CARE

Once a decision about the nature of therapy has been made, how that decision is implemented can have a profound influence on the outcomes of treatment. While decisions about the selection of specific treatment options may occur simultaneously with the implementation of some aspects of care, the processes of design and implementation can be separated. While nurses, patients, and families rarely exercise control over the design of therapy, they do play an important role in its implementation.

Some patients and families were active participants, and staff expected and relied on this involvement.

Several clinic patients received specific instructions about their treatment. One man was given his pills, but was not supposed to start taking them until he got the results of his blood test. Another patient was asked to take his temperature at home and to call if it was more than 37.5° C. The wife of a third patient with a skin infection was asked to observe the rash to see if it was spreading.

Often, patients and families voluntarily become active participants. Patients question nurses about drug administration when they think they may not be getting the correct drug or dose. Many patients and families spontaneously report on the side effects of treatments. One patient's wife regularly phoned in the results of her husband's blood work, which had been done at the local rural hospital, and then received advice from the clinic about adjusting his drug dosages. Other patients and families read about their diseases and treatment so they can participate more knowledgeably in the care. The extent of family involvement in the implementation of patient care is illustrated in the following letter written by the wife of a patient:

Dear Dr. Alexis:

Mr. Gulbrandsen has been home for two weeks now, and is progressing slowly. He's been on prednisone, 7.5 mg. daily. He is up most of the day, eating three meals and feeling much stronger. When he is by himself, with no company around, his teeth complaints are still very real to him. His only other complaints are the irritating running of the nose whenever he eats a meal. He is becoming a bit more communicative and does not stare into space for lengthy periods of time. Please let me know when dental appointments can be set up as the dentist will have to be notified re a penicillin shot before he does any work on him. Hopefully, the blood test he had on Friday was okay. Will see you next Monday.

Other families participate by undertaking complicated treatment regimens in the home. One daughter cared for her mother's deteriorated chest wall at home: she said she did the dressings herself because she thought it would be too hard on the nurses. Another daughter was even willing to take her father home on a respirator.

While most of such active participation enhances the delivery of care, difficulties arise if the treatment plan is incorrectly implemented. For example, one patient reversed the sequence of her chemotherapy drugs and another took his pills all at once instead of spacing them out. Community nurses play an important role in detecting such errors.

Some patients and families actively seek improved care when they perceive inadequate treatment. One patient was convinced her physician was not monitoring her disease properly, so one day she walked into an outpatient clinic and asked to be seen. A mother in a remote settlement also used her own initiative to obtain treatment for her infant son:

The mother said she first suspected something was wrong with her son when he was about three months old because he was having difficulty breathing. She took the baby to the nurse, but the nurse didn't think there was anything wrong. The baby got worse, so the mother took the baby to another nearby settlement. The nurse there agreed there was a problem and sent the baby to the regional hospital. A congenital heart defect was subsequently diagnosed in the child.

While some patients and families are active participants in implementing care, others remain essentially passive. Some believe that they do not have any choice but to accept therapy, and as a result let health personnel implement whatever treatment they want. One such patient, who was extremely quiet, said his physicians gave him a lot of information about his disease and treatment, but he did not ask any questions. Such patients are a source of frustration to health personnel who expect young, alert patients to be active participants in their own care. However, many patients coming to outpatient clinics do not share that expectation. One patient said he was surprised when the staff asked him to report on his experiences with the treatment; he thought they were supposed to tell him what would be happening.

Patients who do not participate in their own care by reporting symptoms can get into difficulty. For example, one woman who had been "feeling terrible" for four weeks did not phone her outpatient clinic. She fainted in an elevator when coming in for her blood work, but still waited until her regular visit the next day to tell the doctor about her symptoms. Such behavior was strongly discouraged by staff, who want patients to phone and let them know what is happening.

Health personnel generally expect that patients and families will be active participants in the implementation of care. Once the patient has made a commitment to a particular course of therapy, there is a further expectation that the patient will remain actively involved. However, not all patients meet this expectation. While there are patients whose spirit "gets them over the hump," there are others who abandon treatment because they do not have the inner resources to persevere.

A patient's decision to withdraw from treatment has a high impact on health professionals, especially if the patient returns for treatment after deterioration has occurred.

> *The nurse described a young woman with cancer who refused further treatment at a time when she felt quite well. However, when she started to get worse, she wanted to resume her treatment. The nurse said the doctors always explain to such patients that, if they go off treatment, a lot of ground is lost. The disease may get worse, and even if they restart the treatment later, it may no longer be very effective. She said she knew it was probably unethical, but she wished patients would not be allowed to reverse a decision to stop treatment.*

In such situations, physicians and nurses feel they have been left to pick up the pieces of what might have been successful treatment for the disease.

Strategies and Tactics

Health personnel use a variety of strategies and tactics to facilitate the participation of patients and families in the implementation of care. For example, some physicians use family conferences to explain and clarify their approach to treatment. Other physicians release information about the disease and treatment gradually so patient and family will be better able to listen and understand what is being said. Still other physicians suggest to patients that they write down their questions and bring them on their next visit. The use of models, diagrams, or analogies are frequently effective in explaining the nature of treatment and eliciting patient participation.

> *The doctor asked the patient what he thought about having the surgery he had just described. The patient said, "It's up to you guys." The doctor replied: "No, it isn't up to us. We can make suggestions, but it's your decision." He gave the analogy of taking a car to a mechanic. The mechanic can say what is wrong with the car, but the owner must decide whether or not the repairs will be done. The patient then said he would need time to decide, and the physician replied, "That's fine."*

Considerable pressure can be exerted on patients to convince them to accept treatment. For example, one elderly woman was convinced to accept treatment by her physician's office nurse who said, "You've always been a fighter; you can't stop fighting now." In another situation, a physician was consulted by a colleague who was having difficulty convincing one of his patients to have surgery for cancer:

> *Over his lunch hour the consultant went to the patient's home. He described what happened at X-ray rounds. "She almost dropped when I appeared at her door." He tried to convince her to have the surgery, but she said that if it's her time, it's her time. He countered by saying that God didn't mean for people to contribute to their own death by not accepting treatment. He then stated, "She expected me to give her a pressure job, but I didn't." The surgeon who had referred the patient added he hadn't pressured her either. He said he would phone her in a week to find out her decision.*

Although these physicians did not perceive themselves as pressuring the patient, others frankly admit they "get tough" with patients who are not following the prescribed treatment. Such tough bargaining is most likely to occur when the patient has a potentially curable disease. If such tactics are ineffective, procedures are sometimes modified to be less extensive for patients who might otherwise refuse all treatment.

Nurses and families also apply social pressure to convince patients to continue their treatment. For example, in a remote settlement, nurses enlisted the aid of community elders in convincing patients to continue treatment. In another instance, an elderly woman agreed to a mastectomy only after her children convinced her that she would not live to see her grandchildren grow up unless she had the surgery. In the face of such social pressure, it is the rare patient who does not give in and agree to participate.

CONCLUSION

Generally speaking, health professionals have a wider repertoire of strategies and tactics for gaining control over treatment decisions than do patients or families. The health care system is structured to ensure that health professionals maintain this upper hand. As a result, patients and families rarely control the design of treatment. Their lack of experience in the health care system places them at a decided disadvantage. However, when health professionals value and encourage their involvement in the decision making process, patients and families are more likely to achieve some control over the design of therapy.

While health professionals do not necessarily welcome patient and family involvement in treatment decision making, they generally expect, and in fact require, patient and family participation during the implementation of care. Patients and families need to recognize that nonparticipation represents an effective strategy for gaining control over treatment decisions.

Based on their previous experiences with treatment decision making for life-threatened patients, most health professionals expect few, if any, patients or families to want involvement in the decision making process. Even if the health professional encounters a patient or family who desires such control, two widely held assumptions tend to prevent the professional from encouraging this involvement. The first assumption is that patients and families have insufficient knowledge to participate; and the second is that, if they do become involved in decision making, they will sustain irreparable psychological damage.

While it is true that many patients and families prefer to delegate control over the design of treatment to health professionals, our data suggest that there are patients and families for whom it is important to have some degree of control. Further, it remains to be seen if these two assumptions are in fact valid. Health professionals need to recognize the danger of using a single bad experience of involving a patient or family in decision making as a generalization to apply to all subsequent patients and families encountered in their practice. Perhaps the real challenge is to discover effective ways of fostering such involvement rather than negating its importance.

5

KNOWLEDGE AND INFORMATION

Knowledge and information are the substance of life–death decision making. The acquisition of knowledge to guide decision making is an activity particularly valued by physicians. The health care system endorses this activity by requiring physicians to seek advice from their colleagues in complex cases. Further, the division of physicians into specialty groups fosters the development of bodies of experiential knowledge about the diagnosis and treatment of specific diseases.

In the process of decision making, a wide variety of information is also sought. The availability, accessibility, and reliability of such information determines its actual usefulness in decision making. Health professionals are responsible for acquiring the information related to diagnosis and treatment, and can withhold or release this information as they choose. Access to knowledge and information constitutes the power base from which the health professional's control over life–death decision making emanates.

KNOWLEDGE

The knowledge used in life–death decision making includes scientific fact and rationale, as well as personal experience and opinion. Basic knowledge is gained through professional education, and provides the physiological rationale for treatment decisions. Physicians are expected to keep their knowledge current by reading professional literature. Citing of statistics from recently reported studies is a regular feature in rounds, and such knowledge is used in planning treatment. The expectation that one's knowledge should be up-to-date is rigorously applied to young interns and residents.

In rounds, the cardiologist described the results of a study about patients with ventricular fibrillation, which were reported in a recent journal article. He recounted the findings of the study, and then turned to the chief resident and said, "But of course, I'm sure you've already read that." The chief resident asked which journal the article was in, and the cardiologist said, "Oh, yesterday's." They all laughed at this. The cardiologist remarked that the chief resident should really keep up with his reading.

At times, being up-to-date leads to a game of one-upmanship among the housestaff or between housestaff and attending physicians. Housestaff who hold the upper hand in this game become enthusiastic, while those who do not become dejected. The resident with a good knowledge base is generally viewed as an asset.

The attending doctor was telling the nurse about their management of a complex case over the weekend. He praised one of the residents, saying he had been a great help. The attending doctor jokingly said, "I know some of the causes of hypercalcemia, but he can rhyme off 26 causes of hypercalcemia in alphabetical order, in order of priority, or in any other order you want." He added that this fellow was one of the greatest residents they had.

At times even experienced physicians go back to the literature, particularly when they are baffled by a complex case. For example, one surgeon spent most of a night searching through his journals after operating on a patient only to find that nothing was wrong. The surgeon described this patient as a "real puzzle."

EXPERIENTIAL KNOWLEDGE

Experiential knowledge plays an important role in planning therapy for the seriously ill patient. In some cases there is simply no scientific knowledge available, so clinical judgement based on previous experience has to be used. For example, with rarely seen life-threatening conditions there are usually not enough cases to develop a scientific basis for treatment.

The physician's specialty area determines the types of experiences he has, and therefore influences his knowledge base and treatment decisions.

The hematologist said physicians in his specialty think it's better not to give patients aspirin because of its effect on blood platelets. They would prefer to give patients some other analgesic. But, he added, "There are a lot of surgeons around who will say they've been operating for years and never had any problems as a result of giving patients aspirin."

Previous cases the physician has experienced in practice often influence how therapy is designed for current patients. One successfully treated case might lead to formulation of a protocol, while one unsuccessfully treated case might lead to future avoidance of that treatment approach.

During cardiology rounds, a heart patient was discussed. Apparently the previous night the patient developed hiccoughs and the resident gave him chlorpromazine. The cardiologist remarked that he didn't like to give people who had an acute myocardial infarction this drug or any of the other phenothiazines. He recounted the case of a patient who had received chlorpromazine only to develop ventricular arrhythmia, and die shortly after. The cardiologist said he didn't know whether or not the two events were related, but there was a very close association. The resident said the patient hadn't developed any complications, but he would keep this in mind the next time he treated a similar case.

Attending physicians realize their residents can make errors in judgement simply because they have never "seen" a patient with a particular condition. Residents also recognize this danger, and frequently ask the attending doctors, "Have you ever seen a case where...?" Some experiential knowledge is developed within particular treatment settings, and physicians are frequently heard to say: "The experience on this unit is..." The recital of particular cases and their outcomes is a frequent occurrence during rounds.

Previous experiences with a disease or treatment also influence the willingness of patients and families to continue or stop treatment. One male patient stated that he was quite willing to have surgery for his cancer because his wife had had surgery for her cancer and had been cured. A family whose son was unconscious and quadriplegic after a diving accident hoped their son would survive because one family member had had a spinal fracture and survived. Another family requested that treatment be stopped when their mother suffered a brain hemorrhage because they had a friend with a similar condition who had sustained serious brain damage. When participating in decision making, patients and families generally rely on experiential knowledge gained from family and friends. If no family member has experienced a similar disease or treatment, the family is at a disadvantage and has to learn about the disease and treatment.

DELIBERATE ACQUISITION OF KNOWLEDGE

When health professionals think their knowledge is insufficient to handle the care of a seriously ill patient, they usually consult their colleagues. This is often accomplished through formal consultation. For example, the following request for consultation from the oncology (cancer) service was found on a patient's chart: "Brain scan suggestive of cerebral metastases (spread of cancer to the brain). Left lung density on X-ray proved to be poorly differentiated cancer. See results of needle biopsy. Please advise re management." Physicians in the consulting specialty assess such patients, leave suggestions regarding treatment on the patient's chart and discuss their advice with the patient's attending physician.

Certain types of consultations occur regularly and are expected. For example, a neurologist is consulted for an opinion on management with all cases of suspected brain damage. A "complex case" might lead the attending physician to consult up to a dozen different specialists. On some specialized units, hospital policy requires attending physicians to consult specialists before undertaking certain types of high risk treatment. While in most situations consultants are asked to provide specific advice in planning curative and palliative trials, at times they are asked to assist in making difficult decisions such as a decision to withdraw active treatment. Such requests are not necessarily related to the specialist's knowledge of his field, but rather to his recognized skill in making difficult treatment decisions.

While the formal process of seeking knowledge is well established, there are also many informal processes that facilitate the acquisition of knowledge. Rounds provide an obvious occasion for informal consultation, and certain locales such as hallways and lunch rooms are regular sites where advice is sought from colleagues on how to manage a case. At times, the advice brought to bear in planning treatment is dependent on which consultant the attending physician happens to meet in the hallway or sits with at lunch. On specialized units, certain locales become regular sites for informal consultations. For example, on one labor and delivery unity such consultations occurred in front of a blackboard where information about laboring women was summarized.

Informal consultation occurs regularly among residents, nurses and attending physicians. Residents consult each other when they are uncertain about a patient's treatment; residents consult experienced nurses regarding the operation of equipment or specific techniques; nurses consult with residents when changes occur in a patient's condition; nurses consult with other nurses regarding the planning of complicated care for the seriously ill patient; and attending physicians consult with nurses about the care of long-term patients who primarily require nursing care. Such ongoing informal consultations occur concurrently with the formal consultation process, but usually are not as adequately documented on the patient's chart.

An adequate knowledge base is extremely important in planning curative and palliative trials. Many processes are directed toward obtaining and maintaining knowledge to guide the design of treatment. While the formal consultation process is important, informal sharing of knowledge also plays a significant role.

INFORMATION

The search for information about patients and their illnesses commences with the patient's entry into the health care system. The patient who becomes seriously ill or develops a sudden complication usually undergoes multiple testing procedures. Attending physicians expect interns and residents to collect information in a systematic manner in order to confirm or rule out specific diagnoses.

> *At rounds the intern presented a patient he had admitted, a 50-year-old lady with a painful swollen arm, a lump in the axilla, and soreness in the breast on the same side. The intern was about to give the lab test results when one of the attending physicians stopped him. He wanted the intern to explain what he thought was going on with the patient at this time. The intern said he thought it was a thrombosis (blood clot). The attending physician got up and set out on the blackboard a whole list of things which could be causing the lady's problems, including a hidden malignancy. He suggested to the intern that he always order tests within a framework, to confirm or rule out some of his suspicions. The attending physician remarked that some of these results really hadn't helped the intern determine what the lady's problem was.*

At times a deliberate decision is made not to collect certain information. For patients who are dying, routine tests such as blood counts are often discontinued. Some attending physicians emphasize there is no use investigating a problem they do not intend to treat. However, if the physician believes that the information to be gained from a test may alter the treatment, he is likely to order it. Experienced physicians recognize when they have acquired sufficient information to proceed with their decisions. In contrast, younger physicians may cite a lack of information as a rationale for avoiding treatment decisions.

AVAILABILITY OF INFORMATION

In many instances, physicians know what information they want so they can make a treatment decision, but must wait for test or other diagnostic data to arrive. One contributing factor is the time lag between the decision to acquire certain information, and the actual point at which that information becomes available. This time lag can be critical for the seriously ill patient.

> *The attending doctor asked his resident what the patient's pulmonary pressures were. The resident said he had tried to get a pulmonary line into the patient for three hours but had been unsuccessful. The attending physician said it was important to have this information because*

he could not treat the patient without it. He said, "I know you're having problems, but this patient was admitted at 5:30 this morning and it's already 10:00. I'm afraid she may die before we finish rounds unless we do something."

Some specialized tests are only done periodically, and results may not be available for 24 to 48 hours. If specialized test systems are not available in the hospital where the patient is being treated, samples have to be sent to other centers for testing. This usually involves a delay of at least a few days. When physicians realize they must arrive at a treatment decision before results will be available, testing may be omitted.

Another factor that may limit availability of information is the nature of the patient's previous medical care and the adequacy of baseline information in the medical history. For example, a woman with a long-term history of emphysema had had no pulmonary function studies performed prior to developing respiratory failure. As a result, decisions about treatment of this acute, life-threatening condition were hampered by a lack of baseline information.

Pragmatic issues also influence availability of information. In one situation, physicians were upset when two biopsy specimens were lost and personnel had to be sent out to track them down. Lost specimens mean that the test is repeated in order to get the desired information and therefore creates a further time lag and causes additional discomfort for the patient.

Inadequate discharge or transfer summaries also limit the availability of information. Patients are sometimes received at referal centers with little or no background information accompanying them. This means that the same information must be collected a second time, causing further delays in treatment. In other instances, patients are discharged to their home communities with no reports to guide local health personnel. For example, in a remote community, nurses sometimes have to make decisions about treatment without knowing what has happened during the patient's previous hospitalization.

Failure to record important information during the patient's treatment also affects treatment decisions. In one incident, the fact that a patient had received a paralytic drug was not recorded, yet assessments of his neurologic status were being made in preparation for a decision to withdraw treatment. Fortunately, this information was discovered by chance and the assessment postponed until the drug was out of the patient's system. In this case, the decision to withdraw treatment might have been made on the basis of an invalid assessment because critical information was missing.

If information is not available during a crisis situation, health personnel believe that the patient should be given the benefit of the doubt and treated aggressively. In the interim, personnel collect crucial information about the patient. For example, a patient with advanced cancer might be resuscitated in the absence of any information about the stage of the cancer. Decisions about changing the direction of treatment can then be made when the required information becomes available.

ACCESSIBILITY OF INFORMATION

Several strategies are used to increase the accessibility of information once it becomes available. One such strategy is the use of flow sheets on patient's charts. These sheets summarize trends in test results, so they can be easily seen at a glance. Lab results judged to be significant by nurses are often displayed in prominent places, such as the front of a patient's chart or the outside of an infant's isolette. On some units, residents and attending doctors initial lab reports to indicate they have been read. When physicians clearly record treatment decisions in the patient's chart, such information is made more accessible to all health professionals.

At times, information is available but not accessible. If a chart is mislaid, an important consultation request may not get answered. Sometimes the sheer bulk of a long-term patient's record makes it difficult to find information without hours of reading. Much information is passed on orally, and if this fails, difficulties arise. For example, one surgeon did not get a message about a patient's high serum potassium prior to surgery, and the patient had a cardiac arrest on the operating table. Families often have difficulty getting information, because they do not have access to the patient's chart and therefore have to rely on information relayed orally.

In many cases, health personnel become repositories of information and are expected to make their information accessible to others when it is required. Nurses usually fulfill this function with respect to information about the patient's activity levels and emotional state. Residents, who are most closely involved in the medical care, are expected to give capsule summaries of the medical history and progress whenever a new physician comes to visit the patient. In remote areas, the Native health representative plays a similar role because of his long time knowledge of residents in the community. In this way, people who are consistently on the scene store information and are expected to make it accessible as required.

RELIABILITY OF INFORMATION

Information may be available and accessible, but still not used in decision making when its reliability is suspect. Test results are usually not taken at face value, but are interpreted within the context of other relevant clinical information. For example, if a patient exhibits all the classical signs and symptoms of a disease, test results which do not support that diagnosis are deemed "suspicious." Physicians are well aware that test results may be inaccurate. They are reluctant to make treatment decisions based on such information in case they will, as one physician put it, "get burned."

Test information can be judged unreliable for a number of reasons. For example, test results can be too high or too low because of failure of the testing system. Such technical problems can be corrected and the test repeated. Some tests are unreliable because of their lack of specificity; that is, they do not accurately detect the presence or absence of a particular condition. In other words, they may indicate a condition is present when it is not, or vice versa. This problem is more difficult to handle than simple failure of a test system. Some physicians are reluctant to order tests that lack specificity. Others order the test, and subsequently discount the results. Debates over the reliability of test results occur frequently during rounds. Physicians prefer to base treatment decisions on test systems proven to be highly reliable in detecting pathology, such as computerized axial tomography in diagnosing brain lesions. However, such highly specific test systems are not available for the detection of all diseases.

HIGHLY RATED INFORMATION

Health personnel consistently rate four types of information as significant in making treatment decisions for the life-threatened patient.

The age of the patient, both chronological and physiological, is usually the first information sought. Statements of chronological age are often expanded and qualified: "He's 96, but he looks very fresh." Age often represents the potential loss that will be caused by the person's death, as well as the potential he has for recovery. The younger the patient, the greater the loss and the greater the chance for recovery.

The second type of highly rated information identified by participants is the stage of the disease: is it in an early stage, and therefore potentially reversible? Or is it too advanced to be effectively treated? Much initial testing of life-threatened patients is directed toward determining the stage of the disease. Health professionals sometimes have difficulty explaining to families why it is so important to do aggressive testing, including surgery, just to get information about the stage of the disease.

Two other types of information are also highly rated. Information about the patient's previous treatment responses and quality of life are usually sought during the process of life-death decision making. If the patient has responded well to a previous treatment, he may respond again. If on the other hand, the patient has a "bad track record" with no previous treatment being effective, health personnel tend to be less optimistic. Information about quality of life is also identified in the process of designing treatment for the seriously ill patient.

At rounds they described the case of a young woman with a chronic problem which became life-threatening. This medical service was asked to admit her. The attending physician talked to the patient and she told him she was happy with her quality of life even though she had disabilities. In fact, she had written a university exam just the week before. The attending physician decided to accept her on the unit, even though there was very little chance of treating her successfully.

If the patient has a questionable quality of life prior to admission, such information is also identified as important in decision making.

During rounds the attending physician, Dr. Bryan, asked the resident about the patient's level of functioning prior to his admission to the unit the evening before. The resident said he didn't know. Dr. Bryan replied, "This patient's a total disaster. He's a good example of someone who should not have been admitted to this unit." Dr. Bryan told the resident to contact the patient's wife to find out about his previous activity level. The resident did this, and told Dr. Bryan that the patient was seriously ill. All he could do for the past six months was sit in a chair. On the basis of that information, they decided to turn off the dopamine (drug to maintain blood pressure).

Information about the patient's age and stage of disease is usually documented on the patient's chart and accessible. In contrast, information about previous treatment responses and in particular quality of life is not usually so well known in spite of its being highly rated.

CONTROL OF INFORMATION

Health personnel exercise a great deal of control over the flow of information, and can decide to withhold information for a variety of reasons. For example, one physician decided not to tell a patient about the side effects of his chemotherapy at the time the patient was deciding whether to take further treatment. Clinical records sometimes note these restrictions, stating for example: "Information about the patient's neurological status not to be discussed with the family." One hospital's policy suggested that if an honest answer could not be given, no statement should be made. At times, the release of information is not curtailed, but rather is carefully controlled. For example, many physicians gradually release information about the severity of a patient's problem in order to reduce stress on the family and enable them to adjust to the information over time. While this approach is usually motivated by a genuine concern to inform both the patient and his family, withholding information may also be used as a strategy to ensure the patient's compliance with planned treatment.

CONCLUSION

While physicians generally base treatment decisions on a common body of professional knowledge, their experiences in caring for seriously ill patients can be extremely diverse. This diversity fosters the development of an individualized bank of experiential knowledge upon which the physician can draw in making treatment decisions. The implication for patients and families is that even physicians trained in the same specialty area may offer different opinions as to the best course of treatment.

Lack of access to information constitutes a major problem for patients and families. Without access to relevant information, it is almost impossible to participate in the decision making process. Patients and families need to recognize that access to health care information must be negotiated and consistently pursued throughout the disease and treatment process.

Health professionals need to recognize that experiential knowledge is as important to patients and families as it is to them. This experiential knowledge can have a profound influence on the patient's and family's willingness to participate in the planned treatment. Before attempting to implement a course of therapy, health professionals would be well advised to elicit the experiential knowledge base from which the patient and family are operating. Failure to do so can result in conflict and frustration for all the participants in life-death decision making.

6

DECISION MAKING

This chapter describes how treatment decisions are formulated for seriously ill patients. We conceptualize the processes of life-death decision making as a "calculation" in which specific criteria are selected and used to estimate the probable consequences of different courses of action. Given the wide variety of treatment options available, participants use systematic approaches to formulating courses of treatment.

Rather than assessing the "fit" between formal decision making theory and decision making in practice, we describe the way people actually think about situations on a day-to-day basis. Further, we were interested in developing an easily understandable way of talking about decision processes. While participants are sometimes aware how they are thinking through and weighing alternatives, more frequently these processes are buried within the day-to-day functioning of each clinical setting. We describe how people actually make decisions in the care of seriously ill patients rather than suggest how their treatment decisions should be made.

THE DECISION MAKER

The decision maker is the person who assumes or is delegated responsibility for life-death decision making; typically this is the attending physician. The decision maker is usually perceived as having one or more of the following characteristics: the knowledge required to make the decision; skill in decision making in general or particular skill in life-death decision making; the ability to gain access to technology; or status, that is the "aura" of being a decision maker. While some physicians are viewed as poor decision makers, others are extremely influential with their colleagues. An attending physician who is considering a particular course of treatment may suddenly make his decision on the basis of a single interaction with a colleague who is perceived to be a "decision maker." Such physicians are readily identifiable in most clinical settings by the frequency with which they are consulted in critical situations. Usually these physicians have had a great deal of experience in making difficult treatment decisions for seriously ill patients.

PROCESSES OF DECISION MAKING

Health care professionals, patients, and families use a variety of approaches as they think through and weigh treatment alternatives. These thought processes are externalized during discussions in rounds or in conferences with patients and families. However, a great deal of "invisible" decision making occurs. One resident offered the following explanation.

> He said physicians frequently have a lot of worries about critically ill patients just below the surface. Sometimes it took only one thing to clarify all those thoughts and bring them into focus, and as a result the plan of care is changed. The decision might look like a "snap" decision, but it wasn't really. It was the product of careful thought and influenced by data slowly accumulating over a period of time on a subconscious level.

This intuitive side of decision making was only accessible from participants who were able to articulate the process. While we were very much aware of their inner turmoil as they struggled to make difficult decisions, we can only describe what we observed and what participants were willing to share with us.

RISK–BENEFIT CALCULATION

The risk–benefit calculation is a type of decision making in which the advantages of using particular treatment options are weighed against their disadvantages. Together with the getting better-getting worse calculation described later, it is the most frequently observed type of decision making. Risk–benefit calculations may be relatively simple or extremely complex. Simple risk–benefit calculations usually involve weighing the advantages and disadvantages of a few treatment options for one major health problem. The decision about which option to use is easiest if one option has a low risk to the patient's life and a high potential benefit. For example, in one intensive care area, patients under treatment for drug overdoses were automatically placed on respirators during the hours they were unconscious. The treatment itself was perceived to be low risk, yet it prevented a potentially life-threatening complication, aspiration (breathing in stomach contents). Such low risk, high benefit treatment options are likely to receive institutional approval, as does the increasing use of caesarian sections to reduce the potentially harmful consequences of fetal distress. Similar reasoning is applied to diagnostic procedures: if the risks associated with the procedure are high and the information to be obtained will not be helpful in planning treatment, it is unlikely the test will be done. Similarly if a treatment option has a high risk and low potential benefit, the decision is also straightforward; it is simply not used.

Decision making becomes increasingly complicated, however, as the number of major health problems multiplies and the number of available treatment options for each problem increases. For example, for one patient who developed two types of cancer, the physician explained he had to predict which of the cancers would kill her first and then design his treatment for that disease. At times physicians are in a dilemma when the treatment for one serious problem (such as heart disease) has potentially negative effects on another life-threatening problem (such as kidney disease). In such situations, treatment has to be carefully designed in order to avoid iatrogenic complications or death.

Perhaps the most difficult risk–benefit calculation is the 50–50 situation, when the risks and benefits appear to be of roughly equal weight.

One of the residents stopped a surgeon after housestaff rounds to ask about a patient who had developed an infection in an artery after the insertion of a cannula (tube). They were concerned because they thought she might have an aneurysm (outpouching of the artery). The resident wanted the surgeon's advice on surgery to repair the aneurysm, or whether they should just wait. The surgeon replied: "You're damned if you do and damned if you don't." He explained that if you go in and put a replacement piece into the artery, they often don't hold. On the other hand, if you don't do the surgery, the aneurysm is likely to blow, and that could mean lethal arterial bleeding. The resident said that the advice of another surgeon had been to leave it alone. This surgeon said he agreed with that advice.

Another difficult risk–benefit calculation occurs when the risks of treatment are high, but the patient will definitely benefit from the procedure. Opinions often vary as to whether such "risky" treatment should be undertaken.

At cardiology rounds they discussed the patient who is having difficulty because her veins are thrombosing (clotting). They were trying to determine whether or not they should start her on heparin to prevent further thrombosis. Apparently, the hematology service had recommended this. The resident said he was not in favor, "because every time we do something for her we get into trouble." However, the cardiologist pointed out that they needed to prevent clots breaking away from the sites already in her arm. They argued about this until the resident

*finally asked, "You want her on heparin?" The cardiologist said "yes,"
and that was that.*

A risky treatment may be undertaken if it is the only option available to
treat a life-threatening problem. However, in some situations, fears about the
high risk of a procedure can prevent its being implemented, particularly when
the physician is concerned about litigation.

If the risks of a particular treatment option are low, it may be implemented
even when the benefits are not high. Physicians, patients, and families readily
make this type of calculation. Patients may use the "it can't hurt and it might
help" rationale with respect to folk cures while physicians apply the same
reasoning to certain drugs or treatments that they know are of questionable
benefit.

*A patient with cancer of the kidney was seen in clinic. The consultant
explained to his resident that chemotherapy isn't very helpful in this
type of cancer. The resident asked why the refering doctor wanted to
put this patient on provera (a hormone) because that drug would not
help either. The consultant said, "It's not toxic, it doesn't hurt." The
resident laughed and said, "Neither does chicken soup!"*

At times the risk associated with a specific treatment is so low, such as one
chance of complication in 10,000 treatments, that the risk is not even considered when deciding. This is small comfort, however, to the patient who
happens to experience that particular complication.

Inevitably, conflicts arise in the process of making risk-benefit calculations.
Such conflicts occur for a variety of reasons. Certain consultants, such as
anesthesiologists, play important roles as "risk-assessors," and their advice
can conflict with the treatment decisions of surgeons who are focusing on the
benefits to be gained from surgery. Consultants who are familiar with the use
of certain diagnostic techniques such as angiograms may disagree with housestaff
who are afraid to order such tests because of their attendant risks. Differences
in perceptions of the risks associated with tests or treatment procedures are
common.

Patients and families regularly make risk-benefit calculations. For example,
patients with cancer are often aware that a serious infection can be fatal, and
take precautions to avoid such a complication. Patients or families who must
give consent for surgery sometimes weigh the potential risks and benefits of
treatment from their perspective. However, they usually identify very different
"risks" and "benefits" than do health professionals. While physicians rely
heavily on test results, families generally identify the impact of treatment on the
individual as being more important. For example, one elderly man accepted a
surgical procedure which only gave him a 25% chance of surviving. His rationale

was that if he died on the table at least he would not remember anything. Treatments that cause pain or prevent the patient from eating are seen as particularly undesirable. One woman refused cancer chemotherapy because it made her so nauseated she could not eat for days. Conflicts sometimes occur between patients who make such risk–benefit calculations and health personnel who tend to minimize short-term discomfort in favor of long-term survival. Similarly, conflicts can occur among various family members who make different risk–benefit calculations for the life-threatened person.

> *During night report, the evening nurse spoke about a dying elderly male patient. Apparently, there was some conflict among the family earlier in the evening. The patient's daughter wanted an intravenous established because she thought it was cruel to let her father starve because he was so alert. The patient's other child and grandchild didn't agree with her, saying they didn't want the man kept alive that way. The night nurse commented, "So it's two against one." The evening nurse nodded, and added that she wasn't sure how it was going to turn out.*

The importance of being able to eat and to be free from pain are recurrent themes in the risk–benefit calculations of patients and families.

Time frames define the limits within which effective risk–benefit calculations can be made. If a patient is treated "too late," the benefits of treatment can be lost. Many treatments are most effective if used early in the course of a disease, but difficulties arise if an early diagnosis cannot be made. Physicians are reluctant to proceed with a risky treatment before a diagnosis has been established in case the patient dies from the treatment before he succumbs to the disease. However, if a patient's disease is progressing rapidly and death is imminent, treatment may be started even in the absence of a firm diagnosis. When the patient's disease is "moving fast" or when life-threatening complications suddenly occur, the time frame for decision making contracts and the attending physician has no choice but to make a decision quickly.

> *About 15 minutes after the obstetrician had decided to perform the caesarian section, the procedure was carried out. The infant was limp at birth, and there was no spontaneous cry. The pediatrician was resuscitating the baby when the obstetrician asked him how much time he thought they had had to get the baby out. The pediatrician replied, "I think you cut it pretty close."*

Most physicians are aware that failure to make the correct decision "in time" can result in the patient's death.

GETTING BETTER–GETTING WORSE
CALCULATION

The getting better–getting worse calculation involves the use of indicators to estimate deterioration or improvement in the patient's condition. Projections for the patient's future health are commonly referred to as the "prognosis." Everyone associated with a life-threatened patient engages in this process of decision making. Participants want to know, "Is he any better today?" They comment, "I hear he's worse." Such statements are repeated time and time again as each participant weighs the indicators they perceive to be relevant.

Judgements as to whether a patient is better or worse may be based on objective or subjective criteria. The objective criteria that can be used to guide decision making include test results such as blood counts, X-rays, and urinalysis. Other objective factors are picked up on physical examination of the patient. Each clinical area has its own indicators that are critical in judging the patient's deterioration or improvement. For example, in the outpatient clinic, blood counts and weights are important in estimating the progress of patients with cancer; on the labor floor, fetal heart rate and fetal blood gases are important indicators; while in intensive care areas, blood gases and level of consciousness are objective criteria that are continually used to estimate the patient's progress. The value of certain of these criteria have been established through previous research. For example, in one intensive care area young patients with accidental brain damage were maintained on life-support systems longer than older patients, because research had shown age to be a significant factor in predicting prognosis.

Subjective criteria are used concurrently with objective criteria. If the patient is looking or feeling worse, health personnel refer to him as being "subjectively worse." Physicians realize that a patient may be subjectively worse even though "he looks good on paper;" that is, test results indicate the patient is better than he looks. Other subjective criteria become important because they have socially ascribed meaning. For example, in remote settlements, the type of health personnel accompanying a patient during transport is an important indicator; if the patient is accompanied by a physician, members of the community know his prognosis is poor. Similarly, children with cancer know from other children that having to take Brompton's cocktail for pain means that they probably will not survive the disease. Nurses often use the behavior of life-threatened infants as a subjective indicator of their condition.

The nurse picked up the infant with meningitis and said: "Look, there's nothing here, nothing a normal baby does. I thought the baby was going to open his eyes and look around. But when he opened his eyes it was just a vacant stare. The baby doesn't respond to you in any way when you pick him up. What an infant to have to take home!"

Sometimes even an examination of all relevant indicators may not reveal whether the patient is better or worse. Information may be conflicting. Some criteria may indicate improvement, while others indicate the exact opposite. Yet the decision as to whether the patient is in fact better or worse is critical in planning therapy. As a result even the smallest changes may be important in judging whether or not the patient is improving. Health personnel in critical care units, who see so many patients die, are prone to use any positive change as an incentive to keep going.

At intensive care X-ray rounds, the housestaff were looking at the chest X-ray of one of their patients. One resident laughed and said, "This is the first time I've been able to even see his heart." Another resident turned to the observer and commented: "Have you noticed how different we are from the ward residents? Any change at all is encouraging to us." Another resident agreed, and said, "We're always grasping at straws."

When health professionals can only provide supportive therapy because there is no effective treatment to arrest or reverse the underlying disease, the getting better–getting worse calculation becomes the dominant type of decision making. In a real sense, the outcome of the calculation determines whether the patient lives or dies. In such situations, treatment is discontinued if no signs of improvement occur within a specified time. For example, when patients sustain brain damage, health personnel maintain vital body functions while waiting to see if they will "wake up," but discontinue therapy when there is no response or even hope of a response. During resuscitation procedures, the patient's response to treatment during the first 15 to 20 minutes helps determine whether or not resuscitation will be continued. While deterioration is often linked with the decision to discontinue treatment, improvement often results in renewed treatment efforts. In some situations, the patient's past record of recovery influences treatment plans; if the record is negative, health personnel are often reluctant to continue.

Needless to say, the getting better–getting worse calculations made by various participants often conflict. One source of conflict is the use of different criteria. While the family often relies on changes in the patient's ability to participate in activities of daily living, physicians rely on criteria that are usually "invisible" to the family, such as blood counts or X-ray results. So, while the physician can describe the patient as being "better today," the family may be thinking "he's worse because he can't eat." Alternatively, family members may see hope where it is not justified. For example, some families incorrectly interpret involuntary movements of the unconscious patient as purposeful, and therefore judge their family member to be getting better. Generally, failure to clarify which criteria are being used in making the getting better–getting worse calculations leads to misunderstandings. Even health professionals do not always agree as to whether the patient is better or worse.

> *The resident asked the attending doctor whether he wanted to discontinue treatment or do a tracheostomy on the patient. The attending physician asked the resident what he wanted to do. The resident replied, "Do the trach." The attending physician asked about the patient's level of consciousness. The resident said he thought she was improving. He then went on to review her other problems. He concluded, "I guess the only real difference is that when I apply deep painful stimulation, it now takes less stimulation to get a response." The attending physician remarked that the family had asked several times about withdrawing treatment. They looked at the patient's X-rays and shook their heads. The resident said, "All in all then, there isn't much chance of her getting better." The attending agreed, and asked the resident to phone the family about discontinuing treatment.*

Sometimes, the consultants called in on a case make conflicting judgements about whether a seriously ill patient will get better or worse. For example, in one situation a family was told by the neurology service that their brain damaged son had no chance of recovery. At the same time they were being told by the respiratory service that their son had a reasonable chance of "waking up." Nurses and physicians also differ in their getting better–getting worse calculations.

> *The nurse said the baby with meningitis was rolling his head and twitching, and that his prognosis is not very good. When it was pointed out that a neurology report was much more optimistic, the nurse threw up her hands and said: "I told them when they were here yesterday that the baby was seizuring, but they wouldn't believe me." Another nurse joined the conversation, saying that she also thought the baby was deteriorating because he was still running a fever and was convulsing.*

Such differences of opinion between physicians and nurses are common, and are usually related to their use of different criteria.

A specific type of getting better–getting worse calculation is the "death prediction." All participants make such predictions, but often using different language. One wife said of her dying husband: "He won't stay the night." Health personnel used a variety of expressions in making death predictions. Physicians and nurses may use phrases like: "She'll probably be dead in a week," "I think this baby has had it," and "This baby is going to heaven today." Such statements are usually made with emotion by health personnel who are dejected by the course of events. Often these predictions are correct.

While getting better-getting worse calculations constitute a distinct approach to life-death decision making, they are often combined with risk-benefit decisions. This is particularly true when there are various options available to treat the life-threatening problem.

> The surgeon explained that surgery would proceed as soon as the physicians were ready. He said the patient was not getting any better, and they didn't know why. He thought surgery was pretty risky, and that after surgery she might only improve for a few days and then get worse. In fact, that happened the last time they operated. He remarked that they were caught in a real dilemma.

In such situations, difficulty arises if some physicians are using risk-benefit calculations to make the treatment decision, while others are using getting better-getting worse calculations. Conflict results unless the decision making processes used in arriving at the recommended treatment are clearly communicated.

WORK ORDER CALCULATION

In the work order calculation, the risks and benefits of treatment options are weighed against their advantages and disadvantages for the work order. The work order is the established work pattern that health personnel follow so their duties are completed in an orderly way. Within institutions, nurses are primarily responsible for maintaining the work order, and as a result are the most frequent participants in work order calculations. While in most instances maintaining the work order permits the smooth completion of tasks, on occasion such calculations are not in the best interests of the patient.

> One patient on the ward died after receiving 15 mg. of dalmane (a sedative). The patient had chronic lung disease and had also had a heart attack. The patient was not a candidate for intensive care and was being treated symptomatically on the ward. Apparently, the patient had created quite a disturbance on the unit two nights previous. The evening nurse wanted to prevent similar behavior, so she asked the medical student to order a sleeping pill for the patient. He wrote the order, even though the resident had warned him that a sleeping pill could be dangerous to a patient like this. The patient "got into trouble," and even though the intern spent all night trying to reverse the effects, the patient eventually died.

Physicians, particularly those in charge of a unit or medical service, are also aware of the importance of maintaining the work order. Physicians may alter prescriptions to facilitate completion of their own tasks. For example, in one situation when a narcotic was ordered to be given every three hours intravenously, the order was changed after the physician was called every three hours during the night to give the drug; the order was amended to an IM injection so the nurses, instead of the physician, could administer it.

In most instances, however, physicians are primarily concerned about maintaining the nurses' work order rather than their own. Even in intensive care areas, work order considerations can affect treatment decisions for the seriously ill.

> *During rounds they visited a patient who had been fighting the respirator and as a result was started on curare (a drug that paralyzes muscles). However, because he was receiving it continuously by infusion pump, he was now so heavily paralyzed that they could not do the required neurological assessments. The attending physician wondered if it is better to administer the drug by pump or to give it in single doses just large enough to keep the patient from fighting the respirator. The head nurse was present, and said the nurses often pressure residents to order the curare by pump. The attending doctor said he understood it took a lot of time to keep on giving single doses, but preferred the latter, because otherwise "the patient just becomes a piece of meat."*

In many clinical settings, nurses are able to exert considerable pressure to ensure that medical orders are written in such a way as to maintain the work order.

SENTIMENTAL ORDER CALCULATION

Participants in life–death decision making are generally affiliated with either a family group or a staff group. The functioning of these groups is easily disrupted by the stress of life–death decision making. Sentimental order is a pattern of social and emotional functioning that maintains the stability of a group. In the sentimental order calculation, the risks and benefits of various treatment options are weighed against the advantages and disadvantages for the sentimental order of the group.

> *The resident was called to emergency where he examined Mrs. Christie, a woman with a bleeding disorder who had been admitted to the unit many times before. She was in a side room and was on a ventilator. The neurologist had already seen her and had given a hopeless prognosis; she had had a severe hemorrhage into her brain stem. The staff wanted to stop ventilating her, but couldn't find the attending physician. The resident said he would take responsibility for the decision, and told the nurse to stop treatment. At this point the attending physician arrived and called the resident aside. He explained that, "for the sake of the family," he wanted the patient transferred to a ward before treatment*

was discontinued. The resident asked the nurse to resume ventilating the patient again, and Mrs. Christie was transferred to the ward before artificial ventilation was stopped.

In a later interview the attending physician explained he had already seen the patient in emergency and had consulted with the neurologist who concurred with his opinion that nothing could be done. He explained this to the family and they agreed with his decision to stop treatment. Then the daughter requested that her mother be transferred to the ward to die. The physician said the decision to comply was based on compassionate, not medical grounds. He had known the family for years and was aware of some family difficulties. He felt that moving the mother to the ward to die would give the family some time alone with her, which would be helpful to them.

In most cases, a sentimental order calculation is made after all conventional treatment approaches have been exhausted. In the previous case, the physician's long-term relationship with the family gave him information that enabled him to make a decision based on its benefits for family functioning. However, even in situations where the staff's knowledge of the patient and family are of short duration, sentimental order calculations occur.

The staff were ready to remove treatment from the young boy injured in a diving accident. The attending physician said he discussed it at length with the family. The family agreed that all treatment should be removed, but wanted one more day to complete funeral and travel arrangements because they were from out of province. The attending physician agreed to accommodate the family's wishes, and had the boy placed in a quiet room so the family could visit him as much as they wanted.

Decisions to prolong the patient's life artificially for the sake of the family can result in conflict. Such decisions are often made privately between the attending physician and the family, and unless they are communicated to housestaff and nurses, these participants can be left in an awkward situation. While on the one hand the decision to remove treatment has been made, "hopeless" treatment is nonetheless being continued. Unless the basis for such a decision is clear to all participants, housestaff and nurses can experience confusion and frustration. However, because of the highly emotional aspect of sentimental order calculations, it is sometimes difficult for the attending physician to communicate his interaction with the family to other health professionals.

In some situations, treatment is initiated rather than removed to maintain the sentimental order of the family. For example, one couple who had an infant with multiple congenital abnormalities wanted to care for their child at home. The physicians decided it would be easier to care for the baby if his large hernia was repaired, so they proceeded with surgery even though the anesthetic risk was high.

In other cases active treatment is continued to maintain the sentimental order of staff. However, participants generally do not identify their behavior as such. Staff are heard to remark: "But we can't stop now; we've worked so hard on him," or "We've got too much invested in him to stop treating." It was the rare health professional who identified the difference between behavior aimed at "treating the staff" and that aimed at "treating the patient."

COST–BENEFIT CALCULATION

The cost–benefit calculation is a process of decision making in which the benefits of a treatment option are weighed against its monetary costs. Only rarely was it a factor in life–death decision making. Cost-benefit calculations, when they do occur, apply to patients who must be sent to another center to obtain treatment. If the patient's prognosis is extremely poor, and the burden of costs to be borne by the family are prohibitive, physicians are reluctant to recommend the procedure. However, special arrangements might be initiated with the provincial health services commission to transfer patients if the potential benefits were high.

Nurses make cost-benefit calculations when they see scarce and expensive health resources being used to treat patients whose prognosis is hopeless. Similarly, when physicians make a decision to stop aggressive treatment but continue some aspects of therapy, nurses make cost-benefit calculations and consider those resources "wasted."

Patients and families make cost-benefit calculations if they decide to obtain folk cures, either locally or abroad. While some decide that the cost of such folk medicine is worthwhile because of the benefits, others change their minds when costs escalate.

The husband had taken his wife to Germany to get some leatrile for her cancer. The tumor didn't improve, and they returned to Canada. They tried to get leatrile here, but had difficulties. They wrote to the doctor they had seen in Germany and he told them to send a blank check, before he would sent leatrile. The husband was a good business-man, and he balked at this. The wife's tumor became much larger, and they returned to the clinic for treatment.

While this family was affluent enough to afford the leatrile, many families can ill-afford the cost of folk medicine, but in their desperate search for a cure chose to use it anyway.

MULTIPLE PERSONS CALCULATION

Sometimes treatment decisions involve consideration of more than one individual. Treatment that benefits one person may have negative implications for others. In the multiple-persons calculation, the risks and benefits of treatment options for one person are weighed against their advantages and disadvantages for another individual or group. Such calculations are often made by the health professionals who control admissions to hospital beds. If a patient requiring concentrated physician or nursing care is accepted on the unit, it means that other patients who require the same care will have to receive a smaller share. Physicians are careful about the patients they accept onto their services, because they have to balance physician resources across a group of patients. For example, a service chief might be reluctant to admit a patient from intensive care after active treatment has been discontinued if the care will continue to consume physician time.

The multiple-persons calculation is also used when decisions are made about discharging patients. For example, home care coordinators are likely to suggest discharging patients when they know there are other sick people at home who might require admission. Similarly, when an intensive care unit is full, the chief physician must decide which patients are not benefiting from treatment or do not need ICU care. Those patients would then be transferred to provide space for other patients who could potentially benefit from intensive care. Such decisions are not easily made. Physicians said their training, which emphasized doing what is "best for the patient" in a one-to-one relationship, conflicted with situations where they had to balance resources across groups of patients.

While the multiple-persons calculation is frequently used to make treatment decisions for groups of patients, this type of decision making can also be used when only two patients are involved. For example, if the decision is made to remove the kidneys of a patient with irreversible brain damage, treatment is sometimes designed in favor of the potential recipient of the kidney.

> One of the residents was called out of cardiology rounds for a resuscitation. When he returned, he reported that the man, whose kidneys were going to be donated, had arrested in X-ray while having his angiograms. The resident said they resuscitated him, put him on life support, and then took him to surgery to have his kidneys removed. One of the other residents asked him if the resuscitation had been successful. He replied, "Well, partially."

In this case, the patient was resuscitated to maintain blood supply to the kidneys, thereby benefiting the prospective recipient.

The multiple-persons calculation is a major form of decision making used in obstetrics, since the risks and benefits of treatment for the mother have to be weighed against the advantages and disadvantages of treatment for the fetus. If the mother has a life-threatening illness, the effect of treatment on the unborn child has to be considered.

A 19-year-old woman was six months pregnant when she came to the clinic for a check-up after having a brain tumor resected. The physicians did not want to start radiotherapy for fear of damage to the fetus. They decided to wait until the fetus was viable, and then induce labor. This plan was carried out, and the infant was healthy at birth. Soon after the baby was delivered, radiotherapy was started.

If a mother has an immediately life-threatening complication of pregnancy, such as a severe hemorrhage, priority is given to saving the life of the mother. Family members are generally in favor of this approach. For example, a husband whose wife was experiencing life-threatening complications expressed his view on this issue.

He said there was no choice between his wife and the baby. Definitely, his wife had the priority. He said maybe that sounded selfish, and he guessed it was, but he didn't think he could live without his wife. He said, "I don't think that's wrong, do you? We have our whole lives ahead of us."

When the multiple-persons calculation involves only two people, priority is given to the person with the greatest chance of survival or the greatest social value.

QUALITY OF LIFE CALCULATION

The quality of life calculation is a process of decision making in which concern over the patient's and family's present or future quality of life affects the nature of treatment. In the usual course of events, health professionals rarely talk about the importance of the patient's quality of life in designing treatment. However, on direct questioning, some participants were able to identify the impact of quality of life considerations on their decision making. For example, one resident who moved between adult and pediatric settings was able to identify that quality of life factors were considered more readily in treating children with brain hemorrhage than in treating similarly affected adults. Even when health professionals identified quality of life factors as significant in influencing the design of treatment, their decision making behavior was not necessarily congruent with their stated aims. For example, one physician explained his treatment plan for an elderly man with leukemia in the following manner.

The physician explained they were trying to get the patient into bone marrow remission so they can send him home. He said they are not only trying to treat the disease, but they were looking at the quality of life. He said the patient is depressed, and they thought that he would feel better if they could get him well enough to go home.

Three weeks later we found the following note written on the chart by the medical resident.

This unfortunate old man is now being kept alive against his will and at the cost of great suffering. The bone marrow remission is completely irrelevant to his condition and should be ignored. Surely the patient's own wishes and suffering should be paramount at this stage. I am in favor, out of compassion if not out of good medical sense, of shedding all further attempts at therapy and of allowing him to die in some sort of dignity. To be aggressive at this stage would be to treat ourselves if it is anything at all. Relatives, friends, and the patient are pleading for interference to cease.

It was only after the consultant from intensive care refused to accept the patient and recommended stopping all active treatment that therapy was in fact discontinued.

The impact of not considering quality of life factors in decision making can be profound for health personnel as well as the patient and family. For example, one nurse who cared for the patient described above said: "It almost makes you think that a person has no rights of their own; they're stripped of all their dignity." When a patient's quality of life is obviously being compromised by the disease or treatment, nurses and housestaff experience real difficulty in sustaining aggressive treatment.

A young woman with cancer of the cervix was treated in intensive care for multiple complications of her radiation treatment. First, her gastrointestinal system stopped working and she was put on hyperalimentation for several months. Then she developed urinary problems, and ureteral catheters were placed in her kidneys. Next, she developed respiratory failure, and she was placed on a respirator and subsequently had a tracheostomy. Now she has gone into kidney failure, and retained a test dye such that her skin has turned a blue-green color. She was extremely uncomfortable, in pain, and had tubes coming out of every orifice. This morning, the resident and nurse most closely involved in her care did not go in to the cubicle with the others on rounds. They just stood outside. The resident sadly shook his head and said, "There comes a time when the quality of life. . ." and the nurse added, "is strained." They both nodded. The resident said, "If it was my decision. . ." and his voice trailed off. The nurse asked, "Have you talked to the rest of the gurus about this?" The resident said, "It's no use. They never give up."

The next day the same group of residents talked about the quality of life of an elderly man who had been aggressively treated with an aneurysm repair.

The resident remarked, "He's a guy who had a good previous level of functioning, so you think you should go ahead and treat him vigorously. You can cure every system on paper, but he's still too weak to do anything for himself. You can keep him alive forever just treating every complication, but the quality of life . . ." Another resident added in a joking tone, "Don't ask about the quality of life, don't ask that question." The first resident shrugged his shoulders and said, "Well, it's questionable."

While the resident's statement that "they never give up" was not true, it reflects the feelings of helplessness experienced by housestaff working in an extremely cure-oriented environment when they perceive that aggressive treatment is no longer appropriate.

Attending physicians tend to think of therapeutic decision making in terms of risk–benefit or getting better–getting worse calculations. If included at all, quality of life factors may constitute one part of a risk–benefit calculation. For example, the high toxicity of a drug may be seen as a "risk" of treatment that can impinge on the patient's quality of life. In such cases, drug dosages may be altered to minimize the negative impact. In this sense, risk–benefit calculations that include consideration of quality of life factors can result in highly individualized treatment. However, physicians still tend to talk about their decision making as weighing risks and benefits, rather than as consideration of quality of life factors.

Family members are more likely to be concerned about quality of life in decision making.

The family of the elderly man with the aneurysm repair explained they didn't want their father to live at all if he was just going to be a vegetable. They said his whole life revolved around working in his yard and playing bridge; these were the two things in life that gave him joy. Now the doctors were not giving any hope that he would ever get back to what he was before; the best that could be hoped for was that he would be able to sit in a wheelchair. They said they didn't want that for him, and they though he wouldn't want that for himself either.

Other families held similar opinions. As one mother said of her brain damaged son: "I'd rather have him die than be a vegetable for the rest of his life." Similarly, the father of one infant with congenital abnormalities said: "If there's any question at all about the baby's quality of life, I want him left alone."

Conflict can occur between families and health professionals when families raise quality of life issues to caregivers who persist in making risk-benefit calculations.

CONCLUSION

This chapter has described one of the least visible and most misunderstood aspects of health care. With the knowledge of how treatment decisions are made in the care of seriously ill patients, families can begin to make sense out of past and current experiences. Specifically, family members need to recognize the types of decision making processes they have been using, and how these processes differ from those used by health professionals. If families are to assess which decision making processes are being used by health professionals, they must persistently seek clarification about the criteria that are guiding decision making. Even within families, various members may use different decision making processes. These differences need to be recognized and discussed if conflict is to be avoided.

Our description of life-death decision making provides health professionals with a common language for analyzing their own decision making. This language is pragmatic rather than theoretical, descriptive rather than prescriptive. In a very real sense, this description provides a mirror in which health professionals can recognize their own practice. If they choose to use this description to analyze their decision making, health professionals will be able to communicate more effectively both with their colleagues, and with patients and families.

Health professionals need to recognize that patients and families use the same decision making processes they do. The fact that patients and families come up with different decisions is a result of their use of different criteria rather than different processes of decision making. If health professionals are willing to share their knowledge and information with health care consumers, there is no reason why consumers cannot participate in decision making since the processes used are common to all those involved.

Any description of life-death decision making is incomplete without considering the characteristics of the "decision maker." The skilled decision maker recognizes the limitations of the time frame and knows when there is enough information to make the decision. Such a decision maker is willing to take calculated risks, and accepts the possibility of error. The goal is to make the best possible decision given the available time and information. Further, it is recognized and accepted that even the best decision does not always produce a positive outcome.

7

DECISIONS, OUTCOMES, AND ACCOUNTABILITY

The processes of life–death decision making most often result in aggressive interventions, or a judgement to initiate or continue curative treatments. When health professionals are convinced that all available treatment options have been exhausted, they may arrive at a no–aggressive treatment decision. At other times health professionals simply decide to wait and see; that is, to continue existing treatment until further information, knowledge, or technology becomes available. Unfortunately, there are times when health professionals cannot decide what to do, and they waffle between one course of treatment and another.

Since most treatment decisions aim for cure, it is not surprising that the most frequent outcome of life–death decision making is indeed a "cure" or, if not that, then at least a resolution of the crisis. However, cure is sometimes a mixed blessing, because it may be accompanied by iatrogenic complications, long-term disability or disfigurement. Should cure prove impossible, patients and families hope a peaceful death will be the final outcome of therapy. Whatever the outcomes of life–death decision making, participants hold themselves and each other accountable for the consequences of their decisions.

AGGRESSIVE TREATMENT DECISIONS

The aggressive treatment decision implies that health professionals have decided to "go for a cure." Generally, such aggressive treatment is continued until there is evidence the patient has an untreatable problem, such as irreversible brain damage or end stage cancer. Before they abandon aggressive treatment, health personnel must be convinced that further treatment is futile. Even after the attending physician has decided to stop aggressive treatment, colleagues may apply pressure to continue. For example, medical residents are more inclined towards aggressive treatment than attending physicians. As a result, residents may try to convince the attending physician that aggressive treatment of a dying patient is justified.

When a patient experiences an iatrogenic or physician-induced complication, aggressive treatment may also continue beyond the point usually defined as reasonable.

> *A female patient with advanced cancer was resuscitated and transferred to intensive care. The consultant explained that they thought the cardiac arrest was due to an electrolyte imbalance induced by one of her medications, and that by resuscitating her, they were "giving her the benefit of the doubt." Later the attending surgeon saw the patient. He talked to the resident about the patient's condition, and then said: "I'd appreciate it if you wouldn't give up on her too soon; we didn't catch the change in her serum calcium for 36 hours."*

In such situations, there is pressure to continue aggressive treatment until the iatrogenic complication has been corrected. As far as health professionals are concerned, while patients may die of their disease, they must not die as a result of physician error.

Most seriously ill patients who can express their wishes are in favor of aggressive treatment. Similarly, families usually favor aggressive treatment, and will exert considerable pressure on other reluctant family members to accept such treatment. Even after health professionals are ready to give up, families may still request continuing aggressive treatment. For example, one family requested that a dying patient receive intravenouses even though he was unconscious. Most health personnel recognize that family members need reassurances that everything possible has been done to save the life of their loved one.

NO–AGGRESSIVE TREATMENT DECISIONS

Even though health professionals are most often intent on going for a cure, there are times when they recognize that they must give up. However, before they give up, health professionals must also be convinced that every possible treatment option has been exhausted. In some cases, when a no-aggressive treatment decision has been made, there is an attempt to obtain family agreement with the proposed course of action. In other cases, health professionals prepare families for the consequences of the no-aggressive treatment decision, without making them party to the decision itself.

Treatment decisions involving the withdrawal of life support systems are by far the most difficult to make and the most poignant to witness.

There was a palpable hush in the nursery, evident by the unusual absence of medical people; only three nurses remained. The cause was Baby Stevens; she wasn't moving and her color was very dusky. The oxygen monitor read zero; the heart monitor said the baby's heart rate was 60; and the red signal light that means the alarms are off was blinking. One of the nurses went to listen to the baby's heart. She said, "It's really sad, isn't it?" Then she covered the baby's body with a face cloth, leaving just the head exposed. "There. At least if the parents come in she won't look so bad." She turned and explained: "You know we turned off the airway pressure. I turned off the oxygen too. It just prolongs it if you leave the oxygen on."

The implementation of such decisions is usually handled by the chief physician or nurse in an intensive care area, and timed so that other health personnel are at lunch or coffee.

Only a small proportion of no-aggressive treatment decisions involve the withdrawal of life support systems. The typical no-aggressive treatment decision is not nearly so dramatic. Decisions to stop a treatment or not to start one are the two most common types of giving up. Most health professionals recognize that it is more difficult to stop a treatment than never to initiate one in the first place. As a result, when confronted with a seriously ill patient whose condition does not respond to treatment, physicians often "do nothing." For example, parents of infants with brain hemorrhage are sometimes told, "If this were my child, I would not treat."

Family members also make no-aggressive treatment decisions. Such decisions are often referred to by the family as "letting him go." Family members can clearly distinguish between treatment that is aggressive and treatment that is comfort-oriented.

The family explained that they were agreeable with the physician's decision to treat their mother's infection, because it was helping to keep her comfortable. However, they would not agree to any treatment for her heart, or anything that would just prolong her suffering.

When families have discussed issues of nontreatment with each other prior to the patient's illness, they are in a better position to make and accept a no-aggressive treatment decision. While family members frequently make no-aggressive treatment decisions among themselves, such decisions are extremely difficult, if not impossible, to implement if they do not have the support of health personnel. Conflicts arise if the family makes this decision earlier than the health personnnel.

When a patient makes a no-aggressive treatment decision, he usually says: "I'm ready to die." Only those patients who remain alert inspite of the severity of their illness are able to make such decisions.

On rounds the physicians visited Mr. Hathaway, the 85-year-old man with multiple complications after surgery. He was lying on his side, turned toward the attending doctor. The patient said, "Why don't you just let me slip away? I'm tired of all this experimentation." The physician said he could appreciate why Mr. Hathaway was depressed about all the equipment, but "you didn't feel this way when you decided to have the surgery, did you?" The old gentleman replied he hadn't, but added, "I didn't really know what I was letting myself in for, now did I?" He repeated that he was tired of all the experimentation, and while he didn't know what the doctor thought, he was not against slipping away quietly. The physician explained that he would probably be going home, and that he was going to get better even if they took all this equipment away right then. He explained that when people start to feel better they get depressed because they notice all the things that are going on around them. The physician emphasized that Mr. Hathaway would probably be going home soon. The old man was visibly cheered at this, but added: "You'd think this was the army for all the troops going in and out of here."

While health professionals recognize that a depressive reaction can occur as the seriously ill patient improves, they also recognize that when a patient decides he wants to die, there is not much they can do but stand by and see their treatment efforts frustrated.

At rounds they visited another elderly patient with multiple complications after surgery. The attending physician pointed out, after they left the room, that the main problem with the patient was that he had no will to live. The physician turned to the dietitian and asked, "Do you have any formula for helping people get the will to live? I don't know what you do when a person rolls over and decides he's going to die."

Nurses, physicians, and family members sometimes receive euthanasia requests from the seriously ill or dying patient. Such requests are phrased in a variety of ways: "Can you do anything to make death come faster?" or "Can you get me a drug so I can finish it?" Health personnel who are experienced at providing comfort care recognize that such requests may have hidden meanings. For example, some caregivers increase their efforts to provide good management of pain and other symptoms in the belief that better symptom control changes the patient's outlook. However, it is true that even patients with good symptom control make such requests. These are usually patients who say they are "fed up with hanging on." In no instance did we observe such a request being fulfilled by health professionals, who generally expressed extreme reluctance to commit active euthanasia or anything that would look like it. At the same time we recognize that if certain health personnel were participating in active euthanasia they would probably not have allowed their behavior to be visible to others.

WAIT–AND–SEE DECISIONS

Processes of life–death decision making do not necessarily result in decisions to change the course of therapy. Sometimes a decision is made to continue existing treatment until further information, knowledge, or technology becomes available. This may be described as being in a "holding pattern" for a specified time period.

Physicians may say:

Time is often the best diagnostician.

I'm setting my time frame at 90 days.

I have to give this baby the benefit of the doubt for the next 24 hours.

Let's wait two or three weeks and then assess the degree of hydro-cephalus.

The decision is to wait another 24 hours and see what she's like in the morning.

The length of these delays is primarily determined by the practitioner's clinical experience. Such waiting periods are necessary for a variety of reasons. Usually the physician believes that further information is required before making a serious decision, such as the decision to stop active treatment. Often the wait–and–see decision implies that careful measurements will be made in the intervening hours or days to determine whether in fact the patient is getting better or worse.

A 55-year-old patient with lymphoma was being treated with predni-sone. His lymph nodes doubled in size over the past five days. The resident said they would wait and see how he responds to the predni-sone. If it is a good response then they will give him some other chemo-therapeutic drugs.

Sometimes physicians only become convinced a decision to stop treatment is appropriate after observing further deterioration in the patient. On the other hand, health professionals sometimes have to wait to be convinced that a patient's condition is serious enough to warrant high-risk intervention. Temporary procedures may be instituted to support the patient during the wait-and-see period. This is sometimes referred to as "buying time."

Wait–and–see decisions are daily occurrences in the care of seriously ill patients. If such decisions specify the waiting time, and a definitive decision is made at the end of that time, few difficulties arise. However, most physicians realize it is easy to "sit on the fence too long." If no time limit is placed on the wait–and–see period, it can extend indefinitely, making participants frustrated by the lack of clarity in treatment goals. Similarly, if a time limit is specified but then is extended repeatedly, misunderstandings can arise. In such situations, physicians are sometimes accused by their colleagues of being "afraid to make a decision." While in most instances the wait–and–see decision is wise because it enables further resources to be brought to bear in treating life-threatened patients, wait–and–see decisions are difficult for participants to tolerate when they involve watching a patient deteriorate.

WAFFLING

While most treatment decisions imply a definite course of action, there are times when health professionals simply do not know what to do, and they "waffle" between one course of treatment and another. Most participants in life-death decision making waffle at one time or another.

The nursing supervisor asked the intensive care resident about two patients with chronic lung disease who were on medical units and whose conditions were deteriorating. She said to the resident it was her understanding that neither patient would be accepted in intensive care again. He replied that the first patient certainly would not be accepted, but about the second one, he didn't know, maybe yes, maybe no. The nurse laughed and said, "You're waffling."

Waffling often involves a back and forth kind of decision making; one day the decision may be to stop treatment, while the next day the decision is to continue treatment. Such behavior produces difficulties for many participants.

At rounds today they discussed the case of the elderly man with multiple complications following an aneurysm repair. The attending doctor said this patient's outlook wasn't very good, and that if a crisis occurred, they should not be too aggressive with treatment. One of the residents commented, "The family thinks we can't make up our minds." Someone asked what he meant. He said: "Every time there's a crisis we go and ask them whether we can do something like put in a pacemaker, but at the same time we're telling them his outlook isn't good." He shook his head.

Some participants ascribe waffling behavior to the need to "treat ourselves" rather than the patient. A few attending physicians recognized that such behavior could occur after decisions had been made to stop aggressive treatment, and took steps to ensure that curative oriented treatments were not implemented. Family members can also participate in waffling by first giving consent to treatment and then withdrawing it.

The impact of waffling is often greatest on nurses, who are easily caught between family and physicians. When physicians waffle, nurses may be asked embarrassing questions by family members who can readily identify the inconsistencies in the treatment plan. Nurses can also be left in a difficult position if the patient suddenly deteriorates and they are unclear as to whether the patient is to be resuscitated. One nurse in such a situation started ventilating the patient and called to a resident, "Are we supposed to be doing anything here?" When waffling occurs, treatment easily becomes half-hearted.

OUTCOMES

The most frequent outcome of life-death decision making is cure, or resolution of the crisis. Infants and adults are resuscitated and sent home; patients with cancer have their disease brought under control; and a variety of diseases and complications are surgically corrected. Such situations are a source of pride to health professionals and of considerable relief to patient and family, particularly if the threat to life has been great. These events are sometimes celebrated; as one physician said, "If this baby survives, I'm buying the champagne!"

Unfortunately, cure or crisis resolution is often accompanied by iatrogenic complications. The complexity of modern treatment means that every potential complication cannot be anticipated. Untoward side effects can and do occur. Some are related to the failure of health personnel to "pick up" preventable complications.

> The third-degree heart block was not detected by the anesthetist during the pre-surgery work-up, even though a cardiogram had been done. When the patient was given the induction anesthetic for his cataract operation, he went into heart block and then fibrillated. The patient was resuscitated and a transvenous pacemaker was inserted.

Lack of attention to detail can easily lead to iatrogenic complications. Physicians are not the only personnel who can make such mistakes.

> There was a dramatic scene when a young man injured in a motorcycle accident was wheeled to the operating room surrounded by doctors and nurses. Apparently, he had suddenly developed an acute abdomen and they thought he had a ruptured intestine. About two hours later, a very grim attending physician told the residents that the bulb on the end of the patient's Miller-Abbott tube had been distended with 500 cc of dextrose and water. This was what had perforated the bowel. He left

and after a few moments of silence they started to discuss how the error could have occurred, and concluded that the two entrances to the tube had probably been incorrectly labelled.

When health personnel make a mistake, they hold themselves accountable and experience feelings of guilt and remorse. They realize there is ample potential for error amid the deluge of information and tasks that confront them daily.

However, iatrogenic complications are sometimes unavoidable if the patient is to benefit from a particular type of therapy. While attempts are made to protect patients from those side effects of treatment that can be anticipated, some iatrogenic complications have to be accepted as the risk of participation in treatment. For example, the patient who develops one of the rare complications of chemotherapy may be cured of cancer only to die of the complication.

While many patients have their life-threatening problem cured, this cure may be accompanied by long-term disability. Brain damage is one of the most tragic of such outcomes. For example, one woman who was resuscitated after cardiac arrest lost her short-term memory, and her husband had to retire to take care of her. Premature infants who are resuscitated and aggressively treated may also be left with irreversible brain damage. One physician describing such an infant remarked: "He's alive, but there's not much left of him."

Another long-term disability that is particularly distressing to patients and families is disfigurement. Patients who experience amputation of body parts through radical surgery have to make profound social adjustments. Often the corrective surgery required for disfigurement is in itself extensive. For example, intensive radiotherapy for cancer of the larynx is not always successful. Such patients may subsequently have their larynxes surgically removed. Due to the damage caused by the radiotherapy, several skin grafts may be required before the neck heals. Such disfigurement is the outcome of many radical surgical procedures.

For a variety of reasons, treatment of seriously ill patients may be delayed. Physicians may hesitate to undertake "risky" treatment, thereby delaying the therapy. Sometimes patients do not seek treatment even though they suspect they are ill. Other patients refuse treatment early in the course of their disease, only to return for therapy when it is "too late."

One surprising outcome of life–death decision making is that patients do not always die after treatment is removed. In fact, some patients actually improve, if only for a brief time. For example, one elderly woman who steadfastly refused surgery for her bowel obstruction caused by cancer gradually improved even though her death had been predicted. One of the nurses commented: "Sometimes it makes you wonder about modern medicine." When unexpected improvement occurs, health personnel are usually dumbfounded, and improvement is attributed to a number of causes: delayed effects of earlier treatment, decreased severity of side effects after treatment has been discontinued, or unknown factors. Usually unexpected improvement is temporary, and is eventually followed by progressive deterioration and death.

If cure or control of the disease is not possible, one outcome highly valued by patients and families is a peaceful death. For example, when a patient dies, other patients ask nurses, "Did he go peacefully? Did he have any pain?" Similarly, families question physicians about whether "the end will be peaceful." Even when extensive preparations are made to ensure that death is peaceful, there is no guarantee such hopes will be fulfilled. For example, one community nurse's efforts to help a family manage the care of their dying relative were foiled at the last minute when a priest insisted on calling an ambulance just prior to the patient's death.

> When the nurse arrived at the apartment the door was wide open and people were milling around in confusion. As soon as the wife saw the nurse, she said, "He's finished, it's all done." Several female relatives were crying. The scene was complicated by the presence of two policemen, one of whom was in the process of phoning the medical examiner. While the nurse was explaining to the policeman on the phone that the man who died had cancer, that his death was expected, and that the attending physician had agreed to come out to pronounce the patient dead, the other policeman was overheard asking the wife, "When was the last time you saw your husband alive?" The wife, who was sobbing, said he had died in her arms. The nurse in all of this was also trying to restore some semblance of order to the household. Later the priest was heard telling one of the police officers that the patient should have been in the hospital all along, but the family would not listen to him. The policeman sympathized that it must be hard to deal with some of his parishioners.

Needless to say, the community nurse was distressed that her three months of work in preparing the family for this event had been so quickly destroyed. However, the multiplicity of personnel who become involved in such crises introduce many uncontrollable elements, whether the patient is dying at home or in hospital. It is difficult, if not impossible, for concerned health professionals to control all these elements and thereby ensure a peaceful death.

ACCOUNTABILITY

Patients, families, and health professionals hold themselves and each other accountable for the outcomes of life-death decision making. Within the health care system, there are standard sets of expectations that define the roles each participant must play if treatment goals are to be attained. Failure of any participant to meet these expectations jeopardizes the achievement of the desired outcomes.

Nurses hold physicians accountable for their management of patient care, and for their general competency in carrying out specialized procedures. Nurses expect a certain level of performance from physicians, and when physicians do not measure up, nurses are critical. Nurses also recognize that they will be held accountable by other health professionals should they overstep their defined boundaries for decision making or make an error in carrying out their designated duties.

The physician wanted to put the patient on a very potent antihypertensive agent. Nurse Stockton was trying to figure out how it should be given and she called Dr. Block over to help her. Dr. Block told her to go ahead and mix the drug while they were talking, but Nurse Stockton refused, saying she wanted to know what she was doing before she mixed anything. Again Dr. Block told her it was okay, that the physicians knew what they were doing and to just go ahead and mix the drug. Nurse Stockton replied, "You may know what you're doing but I'm the one who's giving it." At that, Dr. Block relented and explained how they had arrived at the dosage of the drug. It took five minutes for him to explain his drug calculations before Nurse Stockton was satisfied that the patient was receiving the appropriate dosage.

Nurses also hold patients and families accountable for following prescribed treatment regimens. When patients and families do not comply with treatment, nurses express concern for the patient's safety and well being.

The nurses discovered that a woman who had been flown to a regional hospital to await the birth of her baby had returned to the village. The nurse suspected that it was at the husband's urging that she returned. The nurse scolded the husband, telling him he was really taking a chance with the life of his baby. The nurse told the husband she wanted to see his wife at the airstrip at 9:00 the next morning because there was a plane that could take her back to the regional hospital.

Physicians also hold themselves and each other accountable. First and foremost, they must answer to their colleagues for the decisions they have made, particularly if the decision has placed the patient in jeopardy or the treatment outcome is less than optimal because of an error in medical judgement.

The radiotherapist was annoyed that the surgeon had gone ahead and performed surgery on the patient with cancer of the larynx before the patient had been screened in the tumor clinic. The radiotherapist said that as far as he was concerned, the patient should not have had surgery. He explained there will now be little response to radiotherapy because of the damage done to the tissues by the surgery. The radio-

therapist asked the nurse to make sure the case was brought up at a conference where the surgeon would be present, in order to, as the radiotherapist put it, "have him explain why he did the surgery."

One of the more formal mechanisms through which physicians are held accountable is mortality rounds, held regularly by each hospital department. In one of these departments the procedure for conducting mortality rounds was the following:

The resident presented the general statistics for the month, the percentage of deaths, the number of cardiac cases, the number of resuscitations, how many patients were admitted, and how many died. Then they went through each death on the unit. After each patient was presented, there was a general critique of the treatment ordered and how it might have been done differently. The words "error" and "blame" were used in doing this analysis. Present were six or seven nurses, including the head nurse, all attending doctors and all housestaff.

During mortality rounds, attending physicians are called upon to explain and defend their rationales for specific treatment decisions. In cases where the attending physician's decisions seem reasonable, he receives the support of his colleagues. However, in those cases where a physician's judgement is found wanting, he can be severely chastised and suffer the embarrassment of a public rebuke. In mortality rounds physicians clearly differentiate between unavoidable death and physician error.

However traumatic the process of having to acknowledge mistakes may be for physicians, they nonetheless rely on their colleagues to draw errors to their attention. When they do commit serious mistakes, residents in particular accept the fact that they will be "boiled in oil" by the attending staff. They learn early in their medical careers that, if you want responsibility for decision making, you must accept being held accountable for how you exercise that responsibility. The two go together.

Physicians also have to answer to patients and families for their actions. For example, one patient was told by his surgeon that some additional surgery he required would not be too serious. However, the patient, recalling his past surgical experience, remarked angrily to the physician: "Some of your prophesies aren't too good."

Similarly, physicians hold patients and families accountable for their failure to follow treatment plans, particularly when it interferes with the patient's chances of recovery.

Dr. Garrett's patient was a man whose cancerous lesion of his vocal cords had been treated by radiation therapy three months previously.

Garrett noted that the man's voice was somewhat gravelly in quality and questioned him about this. The man explained he had done some smoking and since then his voice had been slightly hoarse. He said smoking felt good because, after all, he had smoked for 40 years. Dr. Garrett asked him if he thought the fact that he had smoked for 40 years had anything to do with his present problem. The man replied yes, he did. Dr. Garrett's tone and manner while he questioned the patient clearly conveyed his annoyance.

In this case, the physician held the patient accountable for the fact that his lifestyle was a contributing, if not causal, factor in his illness.

The extent to which patients, families, and health professionals hold each other accountable is a reflection of their expectations. Nurses are expected to provide safe, compassionate patient care. Physicians are expected to exercise sound clinical judgement and to be competent practitioners of their art. Additionally, they are expected to care about patients and families, and to demonstrate this understanding and concern in their encounters with them. Families are expected to ally themselves with health professionals by reinforcing and facilitating treatment plans, and at the same time to provide effective emotional support to the patient. Health professionals expect that patients will comply with treatment with a minimum of fuss, and that they will not engage in any activities that may sabotage treatment outcomes. When patients, families, and health professionals do not measure up to these expectations, they are held accountable for their actions.

CONCLUSION

Families need to recognize that health professionals have a pervasive cure-orientation that inevitably leads to the dominance of aggressive treatment decisions. Such decisions only change in the face of overwhelming evidence that no further treatment will be effective. Health professionals are often gathering such evidence even as aggressive treatment continues. In these cases, it may appear to the family that aggressive treatment is being continued when it is no longer justified. However, health professionals will not give up until there is no doubt that discontinuing treatment is the only reasonable course of action.

Although it may not be obvious to patients and families, health professionals are forced through formal and informal mechanisms to be accountable for their actions. In fact, we observed many instances where professional colleagues held each other accountable, but in very few instances were they held accountable by patients and families. While it is clear that patients and families do have expectations about the behavior of health professionals, these are seldom communicated directly to caregivers. Open communication about such expectations among all participants in life-death decision making would do much to reduce potential sources of conflict.

8

IMPACT ON HEALTH PROFESSIONALS

Participation in life-death decision making has a profound impact on health professionals. Although the nature of the impact varies widely, we identify certain commonalities that call into question some popular beliefs about the reactions of health professionals. They do not emerge as hardened or emotionally numbed by daily exposure to death and dying, but rather as sensitive human beings who were deeply moved by the situations in which they found themselves. They clearly felt the weight of the decisions they had to make.

Of any group of health professionals, nurses have the most consistent contact with life-threatened patients and their families on a day-to-day basis. As a result, nurses are deeply affected by their participation in life-death decision making. We identified three major sources of stress on nurses: the types of decisions made by physicians in designing treatment for life-threatened patients; the characteristics of the settings in which the nurses worked; and the specific patient care situations in which they were involved. Nurses demonstrated several patterns of response to the stress of involvement in life-death decision making.

Participation in life-death decision making is also stressful for physicians. For them the major sources of stress are the processes of decision making, the daily confrontation with their limited ability to control the progress of disease, and the unpleasant task of having to tell patients and families the bad news of a poor prognosis. Like nurses, physicians demonstrate specific responses to these stresses. We found that few support systems are available to sustain health professionals who practice in this very difficult field of health care.

IMPACT OF LIFE–DEATH DECISION MAKING ON NURSES

Decisions made by physicians have a major impact on nurses. Nurses are particularly upset when physicians waffle. When this occurs, nurses are often compelled to make treatment decisions for the physician. In so doing, they find themselves assuming responsibility for decisions they do not feel qualified to make. This is especially true when nurses have to decide whether to resuscitate a patient who has suffered a cardiac arrest. Nurses consistently spoke of the unfairness of being placed in this position. In one resuscitation case involving a 96-year-old man, the nurses described their frustrated efforts to have the medical staff make a definite decision:

> *While the resuscitation of this 96-year-old man was going on, nurses at the desk said they had asked the doctors on each of the three days previous whether they should call a 99 on this patient. More than one nurse had asked the doctors about this, but according to the nurses, "the doctors wouldn't leave an order either way." Another added that she had asked again that morning and the resident had told her to ask him again in an hour. In the meantime, the patient arrested and the nurses had to call a 99. A nurse was asked whether they preferred a more definite answer from the physicians. She said yes, she thought they should be able to say one way or the other. She added that often intensive care staff give them a hard time when they call a 99 on a patient like this.*

According to one senior nurse administrator, waffling by physicians, especially when compounded by a lack of adequate communication with the nursing staff, is the most consistently upsetting problem faced by nurses caring for life-threatened patients.

Nurses are also upset by those treatment decisions with which they do not agree, particularly when they are the ones who have to implement the decision. Aggressive treatment that nurses do not think is warranted provokes the most intense resentment. When nurses try to make their concerns regarding aggressive treatment known to medical staff, they meet with varying degrees of success. In one situation, a nurse questioned the decision to resuscitate a patient with a poor prognosis, but was bluntly told, "Just resuscitate him." Although not totally powerless in such situations, nurses do find themselves in the position of carrying out orders with which they disagree and over which they have little control. Theoretically, nurses can refuse to be involved in treatment plans or procedures with which they disagree, but workplace realities usually preclude this alternative. Not surprisingly, nurses respond to such situations with anger, frustration, and resentment.

The no-aggressive treatment decision gives rise to emotional conflict within nurses. While on one level they acknowledge that the decision to stop treatment may be the best in the long run for both the patient and the family, on another and perhaps deeper level, that decision may be in conflict with their personal beliefs and religious convictions. Nurses working in intensive care units are the most likely to be involved in this type of situation, and it is young and inexperienced nurses, who have not worked through their feelings about removal of treatment, who are the most deeply affected. One new graduate who had worked in the intensive care unit for eight months described her feelings after respiratory support was removed from a patient who had suffered irreversible brain damage:

They turned one off the other day. I didn't agree. I guess it was for the best; there was no point in going on. It was better for the parents if the baby went now in the first week of life rather than later. I think a person must get very callous working here.

The head nurse of an intensive care unit described a similar situation in which she tried to help a new nurse cope with her feelings about a no-aggressive treatment decision:

Head nurse Brown said Miss Flett, the nurse caring for the patient, cried hysterically when treatment was stopped. Miss Flett said she had become a nurse to help people, and according to nurse Brown, could not see that by sometimes withholding treatment we help a person as well. Nurse Brown added that it took almost four years before nurse Flett learned to cope with her emotions.

By virtue of their role as part of the patient and family support system and their membership in a professional group, nurses sometimes find themselves in the difficult position of divided loyalties. A treatment decision may have beneficial effects for one group and at the same time produce stresses for another. Nurses experience considerable internal conflict in trying to sort out whose needs should take priority.

A patient was transferred from ICU to a ward accompanied by all her life support equipment. It was clear that the move was in preparation for a decision to stop treatment. The evening charge nurse was not pleased because it meant extra work. Another staff member was experiencing a different kind of stress. This was her first patient death. The unit's head nurse, Mrs. Barnes, recognized that there was good reason for the decision. If the patient had stayed in emergency they couldn't keep her body very long because of the need to free the bed space. On the ward they could keep her body and her husband and family could spend some time with her. Nurse Barnes said she realized that the unit staff were upset that the patient had been brought up to the ward, but she still thought it was best for the family.

When family and nursing priorities conflict, experienced nurses tend to favor a decision that is in the best interest of the family.

IMPACT OF SETTINGS ON NURSES

The characteristics of the settings in which nurses work are potential sources of stress. Virtually every setting has some special characteristics that, while present to a certain degree in other settings as well, are accentuated to the point where they become stressors. In remote settings, isolation and scarce manpower resources mean long working hours and concentrated responsibility for decision making. Because there are few support systems to help nurses in remote areas, they repeatedly experience both physical and psychological exhaustion.

> *During supper a nurse described a colleague who had been alone for six weeks during the summer at one of the northern stations. This nurse had said that by the fourth week she was going "squirrelly." The nurses agreed this could happen, especially if you had calls every night and could never get enough sleep. One of the nurses said, "It gets to the point where, you know you are going to cry if the bell rings one more time."*

In intensive care units, where space is limited and nurses work amid a constant tangle of people and equipment, tension runs high and tempers sometimes flare. The fact that these units seem constantly overheated does nothing to ease the pressure that can build up to the point where, as one nurse put it, she just wanted to go into a corner and scream. The level of care required by patients in such units is complex and demanding, often requiring the full-time attention of at least one nurse per patient. Such constant attention to the intricate details of care is identified by nurses as being both physically and mentally wearing.

> *A baby with multiple congenital abnormalities became the topic of coffee conversation for the ICU nurses who commented on the heavy care he needed and how he required the total attention of one nurse per shift. They said you just couldn't care for this baby day after day; it got to be too much. One problem was that the baby required so much equipment that you literally couldn't find the baby for the equipment.*

The effect of caring for such seriously ill patients continually is well recognized by head nurses who try to ensure that the responsibility for such patients is rotated among the nursing staff.

The concentration of critically ill patients in intensive care units means that nurses in these areas are usually caring for patients who have a high probability of dying. Once patients begin to improve, they are transferred from the intensive care unit only to be replaced by other critically ill patients. Some nurses have difficulty coping with this repeated cycle. One head nurse noted that when new staff nurses have worked in intensive care about four months they go into a period of depression; if they can sort out their feelings, they stay, if they can't, they leave.

In the palliative care unit, nurses work almost exclusively with dying patients. Recovery is an exception and cure is not an expected outcome. Patients are not transferred; they die on the unit. For nurses in this setting, comfort rather than cure is the goal. Although little can be done to forestall the patient's death, nursing care designed to help the patient die in peace and comfort can make the last days of life worth living. However, such nursing care requires a tremendous daily expenditure of emotional energy on the part of the nursing staff, and at times it is more than they can give.

> The nurse said working on the palliative care ward "gets" to people after awhile. She said there are times when she notices an underlying irritability and depression in the behavior of staff. Often, she said, "You don't know that it is happening to you. You know where patients are headed when they come through these doors. After awhile you insulate yourself and don't get as involved. You're always giving, you're not getting anything back. Eventually you become emotionally bankrupt."

The structuring of health facilities into specialized units where there are high concentrations of critically ill or dying patients produces significant psychological impact on the nurses working in these areas. Physicians can come and go, but for nurses providing direct patient care, there is no escape.

IMPACT OF PATIENT CARE SITUATIONS ON NURSES

The patient care situations that have the most profound and long-lasting impact on nurses are those involving the death of a young person, especially a child or a young adult with a family. After listening to countless "remember Mr. So-and-so" conversations, we were struck by one consistent theme—the patients who were best remembered were almost invariably young. In one such discussion, nurses described the following patients: a young man in his early twenties with disfiguring facial cancer; a 23-year-old woman who was diagnosed with a brain tumor three months after giving birth to a baby; a 17-year-old with Hodgkin's disease; and a young architect with small children. In most cases, the nurses could remember some particularly poignant anecdote to tell those members of the staff who might not have known the patient. For example, the young mother went blind before her death and could no longer see her baby; the 17-year-old with Hodgkin's disease turned to his father and said goodbye just before he died; and the young architect used his last strength to thank a nurse for his pain medication just minutes before his death. These stories became part of the folklore of the unit, and we heard others like them repeated many times by many staff members. Like folk tales, the facts of the cases were probably blurred with time, but one characteristic was not: the sense of tragic injustice that anyone should die so young and that they, the nurses, should be so helpless to prevent it.

Although nurses realize that they are powerless to prevent the death of a terminally ill patient, they nonetheless feel responsible for the conditions under which the patient dies. When nurses perceive that a patient has died under less than favorable conditions, they believe they have failed both the patient and the family. Feelings of guilt and self-recrimination are often expressed. Even though the circumstances may have been beyond the nurses' control, they still feel they have broken their trust with the patient and let the family down.

Most nurses have difficulty coping with death. Over time they learn to control their emotions because they have to in order to function effectively. However, they often remember their feelings the first time they experienced a patient's death. As a result, nurses are usually sympathetic and understanding towards students' reactions to death, knowing that they too will learn in time.

> *Nurse Hardy said she actually had a student who broke down and cried with the family, but she didn't think it was a bad thing. She said it helped show this family that all nurses aren't hardened. At the same time she said staff nurses really shouldn't do that if they expect to retain their effectiveness. Nurse Hardy added that when the student faced her second death on the unit, she was able to help without crying.*

For many nurses, learning to cope with death means learning to hide their emotions behind a "front" that is impenetrable to all but their fellow workers.

> *Nurse Stanley said staff often felt much more deeply than what is indicated by their behavior. Although their comments might sound cold and unfeeling, they were not always accurate representations of a staff member's emotions. Nurse Stanley gave the example of a nurse who appears rather flippant and callous in her statements and yet is a very sensitive person. A few weekends previous Dr. Graham phoned nurse Stanley to discuss decisions that were being made about removing a patient's life support system. He had said, "And the grim reaper's standing beside me," an obvious reference to this nurse who had earlier said something like, "Oh, for heaven's sake, why don't you turn that patient off and get it over with." Nurse Stanley said that statement would not reflect how the nurse was really feeling. She observed, "You learn to work in highly emotional situations by putting your own*

emotions on hold and by not responding to them until the moment is appropriate."

Unfortunately, professional control and the "tough front" it manifests can easily be interpreted by patients and families as insensitivity.

Caught up in trying to cope with their own emotions, many nurses have difficulty talking to patients about their illness or impending death. Frequently they voice feelings of inadequacy. Some nurses admit they focus on other aspects of care such as pain control because it is easier to deal with than the patient's emotions. The majority of nurses believe that care of the life-threatened patient includes care of the family, and this can produce additional stress. For example, nurses find it difficult to cope with families who blame them for the patient's illness, or accuse them of giving inadequate care. In one situation, the nurses solved their problems with the patient's family by having the patient transferred to another ward.

Nurse Hudson talked about a patient who had died. She said the patient's family had been difficult to cope with because they blamed the nurses and the hospital for their mother's death. She didn't think that was fair because the family had not made sure that their mother took her medication when she was home. Nurse Hudson said: "I can't remember when I've talked so hard and so fast to get a patient into the intensive care unit."

RESPONSES TO INVOLVEMENT IN LIFE–DEATH DECISIONS

Attachment is one response to involvement in life–death decision making and is most likely to occur when nurses have known a patient over a long period of time and when an emotional bond has developed. In such situations, nurses may identify with, or ascribe certain characteristics to, the patient. While nurses acknowledge the nurse-patient relationship that evolves from this attachment is rewarding, it nonetheless leaves them open to grief when the patient dies. Some nurses question the wisdom of such emotional involvement.

Nurse Kotter described one of her patients who had died at home, and with whom she quickly established a "special" relationship during the months before; it was almost as if she had been drawn into the family and had become part of their support system. She said it had been a difficult experience for her in that she had invested a lot of herself in the situation. Although she was personally satisfied at the end of the experience, she doubted whether she could do it again and whether it was wise to ever become so involved.

One nurse said she was so upset after a patient died that she spent most of the evening crying. Similarly, nurses in the neonatal intensive care unit became attached to infants whom they cared for over a long period of time, and so it was emotionally difficult for them when such infants died.

Nurses readily identify with patients when the patient reminds them of someone they know, or when they themselves have been involved in a similar situation.

> *Nurse Murphy said she had known Mrs. Kane for years because she had been treated repeatedly on her unit. During this time she had several opportunities to talk with Mrs. Kane's children. She felt she shared a common bond with them because their experience was so similar to her own situation in which she had an ill family member. Nurse Murphy agreed that Mrs. Kane's death was difficult for her because she was making an association between this patient and her own family situation.*

Nurses readily ascribe characteristics to their infant patients. They identify feelings in infants and ascribe emotional characteristics to them. Nurses talk directly to the infants and question them about their health status, worries, frustrations, and problems. Orders for the infants' treatments are written as though the infants' are talking directly to the staff, and expressing their own particular preferences for care.

> *A great variety of signs were displayed around the baby's crib. Some of these read: "Hold me," "Cuddle me," "Play with me," and in brackets under all this "Please watch my diaper rash." Other signs read: "Please position me so my fingers are free to suck and explore," "Place a roll in front of my stomach and let me lie on it, this helps me flex my shoulders and I like it," "Tube feed between bottle feedings so I don't get tired or discouraged."*

Because the infants could not speak for themselves, the nurses spoke for them.

In contrast to attachment, detachment involves emotional and/or physical withdrawal of the nurse from the patient. This response occurs when nurses are experiencing "emotional bankruptcy." For example, when a patient to whom a nurse has become attached dies, she may at least temporarily detach herself from further emotional involvement with dying patients. Attachment therefore constitutes a double-bind for nurses. In order to achieve a sense of purpose and fulfillment from their work they believe it is desirable to develop a close, caring relationship with patients and their familes. Yet, such an investment of emotional energy can leave them feeling depleted and empty after the patient dies. This can then result in their avoidance of any emotional involvement with patients—the very factor that makes them feel satisfied with their jobs.

Justification is a response in which rationalization is used to reduce the emotional effects of participation in life–death decision making. Nurses frequently respond in this way to justify the negative consequences of their actions. For example, one nurse felt badly because a patient's death went undiscovered for an inordinately long time on her shift. She justified not finding the patient sooner by stating: "Even with us making rounds every hour or two, if the patient dies immediately after you've been in the room, then it's at least an hour before you find him." In another situation, nurses requested a no-resuscitation order for a patient who subsequently died. They justified their request by saying, "After all, he was 96 and had a huge inguinal hernia that was probably going to strangulate" and "he was probably full of cancer." The process of justification helps nurses cope with the emotional effects of their participation in life–death decision making by decreasing their sense of personal culpability, especially when something goes wrong.

Working with life-threatened patients seems to take, as one nurse put it, "a maturity unrelated to age." Nurses who have such maturity are able to understand their own feelings, know how to control them, and at the same time be sensitive to the needs of patients and families while maintaining their professional role. The wonder is not that nurses sometimes fail to act in this manner, but rather that they succeed as often as they do.

IMPACT ON PHYSICIANS

For physicians the most powerful source of stress is their participation in the process of making life–death decisions. Physicians agonize over when to treat and when not to treat a patient with a questionable prognosis. In this situation, physicians often "search their souls" for the right decision. Few physicians have any desire to "play God," while younger physicians in particular are only too happy to have the burden of responsibility removed from their shoulders by someone higher up in the medical hierarchy.

How to treat critically ill patients is often as problematic as when to treat them. The following example described the frenzied activity of one experienced physician as he tried to sort out just how he should proceed in a complex case.

> *Dr. Bantry spent almost all morning at the patient's bedside, walking back and forth between it and the nurses' desk: reading the notes and latest results of the blood work; going back to the patient to note how much urine was in the bag, or just to look at the patient; then returning to the desk where he would talk to anybody nearby about the patient.*

Sometimes the stress of treating a life-threatened patient becomes so overwhelming that the physician becomes "paralyzed" and cannot make a decision. He must then rely on perceptive colleagues to recognize his plight, and to help him control his anxiety enough to select a course of action.

Apart from the actual process of decision making, working daily with

...reatened patients is a universally draining experience for physicians. They experience anger and frustration when a patient gets worse, and rail against a fate they cannot control when patients develop rare or unforeseen complications. Always the unspoken question is "Why?" Why does this have to happen to this patient at this time? They are the doctors. They are supposed to know, to be in control. Perhaps the hardest lesson that any young physician learns is that there are some things you cannot know and some things you cannot control. However much the learning of that lesson may diminish the sense of personal culpability, it appears to do little to lessen the anger, especially when the patient is young.

> A patient with breast cancer was presented at rounds. Over a two-week period her X-rays changed such that a two by three inch mass was now visible in her chest. The radiotherapist shook his head and remarked, "Her disease is moving fast." The chemotherapist asked whether the patient was young. The radiotherapist looked at her chart and replied, "Yes, forty-five." "Damn," said the chemotherapist.

Inspite of the intensity of their emotions, physicians seldom discuss their feelings with each other. At the same time we found ample evidence for their need of a sympathetic listener. Usually all it took for physicians to "open up" was for us to indicate our sympathy for them in a difficult situation. With colleagues, however, a silent shaking of the head while staring at the floor was the most frequent means of expressing the sense of helplessness and futility experienced in response to a hopeless prognosis.

> The CAT scan showed blood in the ventricles (indicative of irreversible brain damage). As the picture was displayed on the screen the resident exchanged glances with Dr. Matthews and just shook her head. Dr. Matthews said softly, "The disease is no longer just in the lung." The resident shook her head again and looked down at the floor. Then she said, "I was hoping so much that it was just an infection." Continuing to look at the floor, she again shook her head and repeated several times, "I was just hoping so much. . ."

Similarly, after an unsuccessful resuscitation attempt on an infant with a rare heart disease for which there was no cure, the physician who led the resuscitation, buried his head in his hands and muttered softly to himself, "Jesus. . ."

In stark contrast are the battles that the physicians "win." Here there is a sense of exhilaration, excitement, and pride of accomplishment. The following example is typical:

> Dr. Wellington said of the patient: "he really kept us going all day—it was kind of fun." He described to the nurse how busy he had been,

*correcting this problem and that problem, running up and down stairs
from the emergency room to the unit. During his account of this
experience he was interrupted several times, but each time came back
to pick up the story where he had left off, like a veteran recounting a
war story.*

One of the least enjoyable aspects of the physician's job is telling patients
the bad news about their prognosis and treatment. Physicians find this particularly difficult if the patient is young, the prognosis poor, or the treatment
unpleasant or disfiguring.

*Dr. Fuller said the pathology report showed this patient had a lobar
cancer of the breast; a "good news, bad news" situation. The good news
is that she doesn't have any distant metastases but the bad news is that
"your other breast should come off too." He explained that the
incidence of recurrence is too high to leave the remaining breast. "She's
so young," he said with obvious sadness.*

Because giving bad news is so stressful, some physicians avoid the task,
hoping that one of their colleagues will assume this responsibility for them,
or that the patient will find out some other way.

Interns and residents have special pressures beyond those directly associated
with the care of life-threatened patients. The process of obtaining a medical
education is a fatiguing and frustrating experience, particularly for the interns
who are on the lowest rung of the medical hierarchy. They are responsible for
much of the day-to-day "scut work" on the wards, often work the longest hours,
and yet have little ultimate authority. Much of what interns learn is dependent
on how much residents, their immediate superiors, are willing to teach them.

*The intern said he had a lot of trouble with the resident on the service
because the resident asked the interns about everything they might have
missed. He said that while the resident played a game of one-upmanship, he didn't want to play because he didn't agree with the ground
rules. With the attending doctor, you could sit down and discuss how
you handle the entire case but the resident would just grill you about
what you missed.*

Both interns and residents feel the pressures of the hectic pace and heavy
work load, and they often wonder aloud to each other whether they are going
to make it through the day. The general consensus seemed to be that you could
work 24 hours a day, seven days a week, and still be busy. Faced with an often
impossible task, they did their best, and fervently hoped nothing would go
wrong.

Like nurses, physicians can become emotionally attached to their patients.
They are aware that this attachment may influence their own decisions. Attach-

ment is particularly likely to occur with physicians who have cared for their patients over a long period and have had time to develop "emotional investments" in them, or if the patients remind the physicians of someone they know.

> *Dr. Lodge approached the two residents to ask if he could talk with them for a few minutes. He said he expected Mr. Norton's family to ask him to withdraw treatment and he wanted to know what the residents thought. One resident pointed out that he was not the one to ask because he was sort of biased, having worked with the patient for so long. Dr. Lodge agreed, saying that he was also biased because if it was his father he would not have wanted him to end up like this patient. He also remarked that it was a shame to be considering withdrawing treatment after all the hard work they had put into the patient.*

When attachment occurs and the patient subsequently dies, the physician may avoid such attachments in the future. Similarly, a disastrous experience giving bad news may cause the physician to avoid future emotional involvement.

> *The nurses were discussing why a resident had requested all parents to be taken into the parents' room for an explanation of their infant's condition before being allowed to see their child. They concluded the reason was because of a previous bad experience with the mother of a dying infant. The mother apparently had burst into tears and cried uncontrollably in front of the resident after he had spoken with her. The nurses were convinced the resident was hoping to avoid similar episodes by first interviewing parents in the private room before they saw their infants. The nurses remarked that they did not think the experience had been so bad for the mother, but rather that it had been difficult for the resident.*

Working daily with life-threatened patients, especially when the battle is being lost instead of won, provokes feelings of anger, frustration, and in some cases, despair. For the interns and residents, the process of furthering their medical training is stressful in itself. They work long hours, carry heavy patient loads, and have to cope with the impact of life–death decision making under the additional strain of fatigued bodies and minds. While physicians seldom reveal personal responses during life–death decision making, they are not immune to the stresses of caring for seriously ill patients.

CONCLUSION

The effect of life–death decision making on health professionals is pervasive and profound. The process of making a no-aggressive treatment decision is particularly difficult for physicians, while the implementation of that decision is stressful for nurses. Health professionals invariably become attached to some of their patients. Unfortunately, with attachment comes vulnerability. To protect themselves, some health professionals avoid emotional involvement with seriously ill patients. Other health professionals respond by pursuing aggressive treatment to avoid loss of the patient. It is rare to find health professionals who are able to maintain a warm, personal relationship with the patient and still retain the professional objectivity required to make tough treatment decisions.

Nurses and physicians seldom acknowledge how caring for the seriously ill affects them. Perhaps the need to maintain a professional demeanor precludes this. However, reticence to share personal responses openly with colleagues removes a potential source of support. If health professionals could share their experiences, they would feel less isolated while making and implementing difficult treatment decisions. Perhaps then they would no longer have to pretend that losing a patient does not matter.

9

IMPACT ON PATIENTS AND FAMILIES

The onset of serious illness produces drastic changes in the lives of patients and families. Day-to-day existence constricts to focus on the disease, its treatment, and its outcome. The stress experienced as a result of treatment is accentuated when there are difficulties in communication between patients, families, and caregivers. Although patients and families often respond to life-threatening illness with feelings of fear and grief, this does not imply that they are incapable of participating in decision making. On the contrary, while responding to the gravity of their particular situation, they are at the same time capable of great moments of courage, generosity, and insight. While a few formal supports are available to sustain patients and families during their participation in life–death decision making, the major responsibility for providing such support falls to physicians and nurses.

IMPACT ON PATIENTS

For the life-threatened patient, the process of receiving care can be as traumatic as the disease itself. Centralization of health care resources means that patients often travel long distances in a fatigued and weakened condition to receive treatment. In isolated settlements, patients are flown out to strange hospitals where they may not speak the language of their caregivers, and where they are without the support of familiar surroundings, family, or friends. The complex technology used in curative treatment can also be a source of fear and anxiety for patients; for example, many patients are initially frightened by the idea of radiotherapy. Some patients just tire of what they perceive as "experimentation," and decide that life is not worth living if it means a continual round of treatments and procedures.

The side effects of treatments, particularly those associated with radiation therapy and chemotherapy, are an additional source of stress for the life-threatened patient. The treatments make them sick and fatigued, cause their hair to fall out, and destroy their appetites. Yet, in spite of these effects, most patients accept treatment and desperately cling to life. One woman, who was interviewed two years after completing her treatments, still had vivid recollections of her experience and what it had meant to her.

It took her about a year before the memory of her chemotherapy began to fade. For months after, the sight of an intravenous pole, or a visit to her cancer clinic for a follow-up, was enough to make her tense. She learned that even though you might say you understand what a patient is going through, you don't really understand until you have gone through the illness and treatment yourself. While she was on chemotherapy, she felt as if she was on a roller coaster, both mentally and physically. She said that both radiation and surgery were nothing compared to chemotherapy. However, there was really no question but that she would continue. She remarked that she was still young, and didn't want to die yet.

The disfigurement resulting from some treatments is particularly distressing to patients. For example, one elderly man lost an ear as a result of complications following radiation therapy for a tumor on his face. Whenever he looked into a mirror, he put his hand over the place his ear had been. A woman in her sixties who had a mastectomy spoke about the importance of the loss of her breast.

She said some people might not think it so important to a woman of her age, but she had always prided herself on her appearance. She had been widowed shortly before her mastectomy, and said that having to cope with these two losses at once made her feel pressured and anxious.

Women who are pregnant when they develop a life-threatening illness face the dual predicament of not only having to consider the side effects of treatment for themselves, but for their unborn infants as well.

Life-threatened patients spend much of their time waiting: waiting for test results, waiting for treatment decisions, and waiting to find out if they will be cured. One woman said her wait to find out if her cancer had been cured was like "being asked to hold your breath for two years." Health professionals are well aware of how anxious patients can become while awaiting test results, and frequently debate how to best handle these situations.

The physician said the patient had been told before surgery that the lump in her breast might be cancer. He planned to do the biopsy and surgery at the same time so that if it was benign he would just take the lump out, but if it was malignant he would do a radical mastectomy. The physician explained he preferred this even though it took half an hour during the surgery to get the results from pathology. If he did a needle biopsy in the office and it was malignant, then he'd have to tell the patient there was a two-week wait for surgery. He said patients found waiting difficult and often went to other hospitals for earlier surgery dates.

Patients become upset when they think that information is being withheld from them. They also do not like conflicting information. One patient was angry enough to write a letter in which she stated: "I've received so many different answers to many questions that I've asked, that I'm quite upset about it all. It seems as if no one has either the time to listen, or to give straight answers." Another patient was convinced she was dying of cancer because her physician had not told her anything after her hysterectomy. In this case, no news was thought to be bad news.

Patients cope with the knowledge that they have a life-threatening disease in a variety of ways. One 16-year-old with a neuromuscular disease revealed the following thoughts about his life:

He had been told when he was nine years old that he would die by the time he was 10. Since then they had increased his life expectancy by one year every year. He said they don't say that to him anymore. They let him take one day at a time. He said when he turned 16, he gave up any hope of being cured and now hopes they can stop the progression of some of his symptoms.

An elderly patient recovering from surgery for cancer of the rectum expressed a slightly different philosophy.

He thought he might have a couple of years left. He knew of people who lived to be 90 and 95 and even 100, but he thought it wasn't good to live so long if you weren't feeling well. He said "it would be better just to be six feet under."

Patients who integrate their life-threatening illness into a personal philosophy of life are best able to manage the stresses of their disease and treatment.

Other patients attempt to cope with the knowledge that they have a life-threatening illness by denying or withdrawing from the reality of their situation. They may, for a time, deny they have cancer and attribute their symptoms to some other less threatening process, or try to avoid discussing their illness with health professionals. Eventually, however, these patients cannot escape awareness of their impending death. Having a patient die in the same room is a potent event that produces both fear and anxiety.

The nurse said they have problems placing patients on the unit. She said that some patients and families keep score on how many people die in their rooms. One lady had a patient in the next bed die, and this upset her so much that she didn't get up for her usual walks in the hall. Another patient was put in the space, that patient died too, and the lady became so depressed that her condition subsequently deteriorated. The nurse said the lady would probably have deteriorated anyway, but it really wasn't a good situation.

Given the realities of many critical care settings where deaths occur frequently, patients find it difficult to deny the possibility of their own death. Even for those patients who have been declared "cured," there is always the lingering fear the disease may return. These patients may interpret any symptom as an indication that "it is back again."

When patients are presented with the diagnosis of a life-threatening illness, their whole world changes. They become prisoners on a crazy merry-go-round they cannot control, much less stop, and which at first they cannot even understand. Overnight, time changes its meaning and takes on new dimensions: where their lives once stretched before them limitlessly, time now becomes demarcated by the cadence of test results and treatment protocols. Life is lived from one day to the next, and the future becomes a painful uncertainty dominated by the questions, "Will I get better?" and "How long do I have?"

IMPACT ON FAMILIES

When a family member becomes critically ill, the whole family is forced to cope not only with the knowledge that the illness may end in death but also with the variety of circumstances surrounding the course and treatment of the illness. In remote settings when a critically ill patient is evacuated the rest of the family is usually left behind, often with little knowledge of what is happening to their loved one far away. The intensive care unit is particularly intimidating with its strange equipment, its staff in a state of constant and often harried activity, and the sights and sounds of other critically ill patients. Not surprisingly some families feel threatened, overwhelmed, and at a loss to know how to act or respond. For example, one mother and father were too frightened to visit their child in a pediatric intensive care unit, preferring to maintain contact with the unit by telephone. Other families believe such a threatening environment is potentially hostile and spend long hours with the critically ill family member in an apparent attempt to protect them, wearing themselves out to the point of exhaustion in doing so.

Several factors intensify the difficulty that family members may have in coping with critical illness. Foremost among these is any perceived lack of sympathy or understanding from the health professionals. When family members surrender their loved ones to the care of health professionals, they can forgive almost anything but a lack of human concern and interest. Physical care and technical competence are important to be sure, but of greater importance is the attitude of health personnel.

The patient's wife said her relationship with the surgeon was not very good. She had essentially two complaints: first, he didn't diagnose the source of the infection, a failure she was willing to forgive. Secondly, she thought he was unconcerned about the ordeal they had just gone through. In fact, she said that she had expected more sympathy from him about the effect this was having on their lives. She was more willing to forgive him the mistake in diagnosis than the other aspect of his behavior toward them.

Lack of communication with health professionals also has an impact on families. Family members are unnecessarily anxious when pertinent information regarding a loved one's disease, prognosis, and treatment is not conveyed to them. Without adequate and accurate information on which to base their interpretation of situations, family members may easily misunderstand the actions of health professionals. This in turn provokes distrust and suspicion. When a family perceives that important information has been withheld, they often respond with anger and hostility. This does little to enhance the family's sense of comfort in leaving the care of their loved one to strangers, and may strain relations between the family and caregivers. Family members need to feel that the care of their loved one is in the hands of individuals they can trust. When this trust is not there, their stress is compounded. Moreover, when health professionals sense family hostility they try to avoid that family or label the family as "difficult" or "unreasonable." This further reduces the information available to the family and tends to fuel a climate of mutual mistrust and hostility. The more health professionals withhold information from the family, the more they fulfill the family's impression that information is being withheld from them. As the family becomes more resentful and more openly hostile toward caregivers, they fulfill the caregivers' perceptions that they are a "problem" family.

A breakdown in communication between the family and health professionals is particularly devastating if the family senses that caregivers do not value information that the family is trying to provide. In several instances, family members tried to convince health personnel that their relative was critically ill, but were not believed. These family members described their frustration in trying to get health professionals to take their concern seriously. In such cases, family members have to be so persistent that caregivers are compelled to listen to them.

Changes in physical or mental status associated with disease are an additional source of stress for families. They become especially concerned by the patient's lack of appetite or inability to eat, and seem to use this as a standard against which to judge a patient's progress or lack of it. Changes in mental status are particularly important to the family; when a patient becomes confused or unconscious, the family becomes concerned that they may never again be able to communicate with their loved one.

When the family becomes aware that their loved one is getting worse, the impact is usually intense. The classic symptoms of the grief response are evident, expressed by family members in their own private ways. Some families are able to grieve openly for the dying family member and at the same time still show support and concern for each other.

> *The resident said the parents had been told that the baby had hemorrhaged into his head and would not live. When the parents entered the nursery they went to the foot of the isolette where the father put his arm around the mother's waist. They stood at the baby's feet and just stared at the baby. The mother was crying and the father had tears in his eyes. A stool was brought for the mother and she sat and looked at her son for some time. Then she put her hand through the porthole and stroked the baby's leg for a few moments before she broke down completely. The parents stayed about 15 minutes and then left. As they went out, the mother kept looking back for one more view of her son.*

Other families respond with less visible emotions, as did these parents who had just been informed that their daughter had sustained a cerebral hemorrhage:

> *The resident was trying to rouse the child by trying to get her to open her eyes and to look at her father. Almost desperately, he said to her: "Come on, open your eyes and look at your Dad. He sure would like it if you'd look at him." But there was no response. The father called her name, again there was not response. The mother entered and stood at the end of the bed, giving no visible sign of emotion. The parents only stayed a minute or so longer and then left. The resident noticed they had left when he looked up from writing his notes, commented to the nurse: "Are they gone already? I thought they would stay a little longer." The nurse replied: "They've just learned about it and they're very upset."*

Some health professionals are more sensitive than others to individual differences in families' responses to a loved one's fatal illness.

For family members, the grief associated with the loss of a loved one is overwhelming, and gives rise to feelings of being unable to cope with the situation. Still other family members believe they will somehow be given the strength to carry the burden.

The daughter said things were not going very well at all. Apparently, her mother had not eaten normally since last Wednesday. The daughter was maintaining a calm exterior as she talked, but her tone indicated that she was upset. She said this had been going on for six weeks. When a person was taking so long to die, she wondered whether an overdose of some drug would be a good idea. She said if she knew that her mother was not in pain, it would ease her mind. She also said she found her mother's gurgling in her throat very distressing. But she added that people were not given burdens without also being given the strength to carry them.

Many families experience difficulty working out their role in caring for the dying family member. Often they do not know what to do or how to do it, and sometimes the dying person's confusion or irritability compounds the problem, making the family feel unwanted and unneeded at a time when they desperately need to do something.

The family wanted to do something for their dying mother, and were asking the nurses for advice. A nurse who was with the patient said she told the family there was nothing they could do. The doctor asked, "But isn't there something?" The nurse said the patient wouldn't let the family do anything; moreover, the family members are really afraid to touch her. The nurse wondered if the patient wasn't taking things out on the family. At one point family members were so upset they were in tears in the hall outside the patient's room.

When a dying family member is cared for in the home, the family faces additional stress. They provide the minute to minute nursing care with no change of shift to relieve them. Nonetheless, some families seem to draw strength from the fact that they are providing loving care in a way that health professionals cannot.

The daughter said they wanted to have her father at home rather than in the hospital even though it was hard on them; her mother often did not sleep nights. She said that she had stayed up until about one in the morning, but then she had gone to sleep and her mother had taken over. The family is turning the father every hour, and in the morning a brother comes down to bathe and shave him. While doing the care, the wife and daughter were hugging and kissing the patient, even though he was unconscious and did not respond.

Families who care for the dying patient at home are intimately aware of their loved one's decline and cannot hide from the fact that death is approaching.

Participation in the care of the life-threatened patient has an intense impact on family members. The pattern of their daily lives is disrupted as they visit the loved one in the hospital or provide care at home. Their goals, hopes, dreams, and plans for the future have to be restructured to exclude the dying family member. Sources of past strength, comfort, and support, such as a father or mother, now need the support of their sons and daughters. For some children, this seems to be a last painful step toward becoming an adult. For others, such as a husband or wife, there is the fear of being alone where previously so much was shared. A part of the self is being lost with the loved one. For parents of children, there is the feeling that somehow they have failed to protect their child from the ultimate hazard. For parents of infants and prematures, there is the sorrow over the loss of someone they have never known and never will know, for all that might have been and yet now can never be.

SUPPORT SYSTEMS

Relatively few support systems are available to sustain patients and families during their involvement in life–death decisions. Those that are fall into one of two types, formal and informal. Formal support systems are standardized approaches, and are officially recognized components of the health care system. Informal support systems represent the more spontaneous and situational types of support that are not part of the official structure of health care. The effectiveness of either support system depends on the quality of the relationship that has been established between individuals involved in life–death decision making, and upon the sensitivity and ability of those individuals to extend themselves to others in a meaningful way.

FORMAL SUPPORT SYSTEMS

A number of formal support systems are used by patients and families in institutional settings. The pastoral care worker serves an important role in helping patients verbalize their feelings, and in helping patients and families talk to each other openly about the patient's prognosis. Although pastoral care workers sometimes think the support they provide is inadequate, patients and staff perceive that such support is helpful, primarily because of the caring manner in which it is offered.

In the pediatric setting, the child support program plays a role similar to pastoral care in the adult setting. Child support workers provide emotional care to the child and family. Initially, the child has priority. The goal is to help the young patient cope with painful treatments, the progression of illness, and the gradually dawning realization that recovery will never happen. When the child becomes too ill to be aware of the surroundings, the priority shifts to the parents and helping them cope with their child's impending death. Child support workers believe it is their role to be there when children need them, no matter what the hour or reason.

A worker described a boy who died several months previous. This boy had had several medications, but was still awake at 12:30 a.m., when the staff phoned to ask her to come and see him. When she arrived at the hospital, he immediately confronted her with, "Why did you come?" She told him that there was another little girl she had to come and see, and that she thought she would just pop down the hall to see him, too. She asked him if he would like her to read him a story and stay with him for awhile. Before going to sleep, he asked if the little girl was going to need her the next night. She said no, but she could come and see him if he needed her. So, she did come again the next night, and a few hours later the little boy died in his sleep.

While institutional settings do provide some formal supports for patients and families, even these limited resources are not available in the community.

INFORMAL SUPPORT SYSTEMS

Patients are often a major source of support for each other, either individually or in groups. In one setting, patients with cancer formed a support group where they shared information about how to cope with their treatments and the symptoms of their illness. The group also served an important function by providing an accepting and supportive environment for sharing feelings that were difficult to express to health professionals or family members

One man explained how group members had formed such close bonds with each other. In the group they shared information about their reactions to drugs and their aches and pains. The group gave them a chance to compare notes and to tell staff about things they would like to see changed. One of the helpful aspects was that on a bad day, you could phone another member of the group to talk. Sometimes you would get concrete advice, other times just talking could be comforting. One of the ladies said, "Often you feel a need to talk about what is happening to you, but you don't feel you can share that with your family." Others said, if you share concerns with your family, they feel sorry for you, which is something you don't need.

Children as well as adults provide support for each other when they sense that another child is in pain or having difficulty with his emotions.

One of the nurses said Jimmy was a sensitive, gentle child. She recalled an incident when another boy in the same room with him was diagnosed with diabetes, and was learning to give himself insulin injections. He cried when he gave his first injection and Jimmy said to him, "I know, I cried the first time I had a needle too—it's alright."

Staff recognize the support patients can offer to each other and sometimes incorporate this into their own patient support strategies. In one clinic an informal support group sometimes emerges when several people are receiving regular treatments at the same time.

Nurse Whitman thought in many ways it was good to have so many people receiving injections at once because it seemed like the group offered support to each other. One person would say, "Oh, is this your first time getting an injection?," and another one would say, "Well, you know, these injections aren't so bad because if it weren't for them, I wouldn't be here." Nurse Whitman emphasized that she thought this support was very important.

The day-to-day role of providing support to families frequently falls to nursing staff. Nurses are keenly aware of the importance of this role and they worry about which strategies will be most helpful in providing support. One of the most difficult decisions nurses have to make is when to notify family members that a loved one is dying.

A patient was deteriorating quite rapidly and the nurse who was taking care of her asked the nurse at the desk whether they should call the family. The nurse at the desk said, "Either they're going to fall apart now or they're going to fall apart later. It's just a matter of how much of their energy is involved." She was concerned that if called now, the family would rush down and there would be a big scene that could go on for a number of hours. Whereas, if they arrived later it would be less emotionally draining. She said they were really caught between these alternatives: calling the family now or calling them later.

When a patient is dying, nurses believe it is important for family members to have the support of staff they know, rather than having to cope with their grief in the presence of strangers.

The staff of one unit was relieved that a long-term patient of theirs had been admitted to their unit before she died. When her husband came to visit at least he knew the staff. The staff emphasized that at a time like this it was important for the family not to be among strangers.

It is often the most simple, yet deeply personal gestures that provide the most touching and meaningful examples of family support by health professionals.

The parents returned after the baby died and asked to see the baby again, so the nurse accompanied them to the morgue. On the way she had some misgivings about the request because she was afraid the morgue attendant would just put the baby on a slab and that it would be very hard on the parents. Instead, she said the attendant was a remarkably sensitive individual, who had foreseen her concern. He had drawn the curtains all around the baby and placed her in a little bassinet with blankets. The nurse said as she was saying goodbye to the parents, she told them how sorry everyone in the nursery was about what had happened. The parents thanked the nurse for all the support they had given.

Health professionals provide informal support to patients and families by such simple human gestures as holding a hand, staying with them when they cry, recognizing their outbursts of anger and frustration for what they are, and sometimes just by keeping a silent vigil with them through the long lonely hours of the night.

CONCLUSION

Once patients and families become involved in life–death decision making, there is no escaping its impact. Irrespective of age, social position, or type of disease, the experience has long lasting implications. Life-threatened patients are forced to confront their own mortality sooner and more intimately than they expect. The family will never forget their experiences during the treatment of a life-threatened loved one. Years later they will still recall details of the treatment process and how these affected them.

Given the intensity of the impact on patients and families, it is surprising that so few support systems exist. Emotional support is left to health professionals who are already functioning under considerable stress themselves. Perhaps one of the most glaring needs in health care is for the development of more extensive systems of ongoing and long-term support for life-threatened patients and their families.

10

CASE STUDIES

In the previous chapters we have presented the major categories that describe the world of life–death decision making. In order to achieve conceptual clarity, these descriptive categories were abstracted from their social context and presented separately to define their essential properties. However, in the real world of life–death decisions, the boundaries between categories may not be so clear. The analytic system we developed to help us understand what happens when treatment decisions are made for patients with life-threatening illnesses imposes an artificial order on what in reality is a much more complex world.

We selected two case studies to illustrate the complexity of life–death decision making. The first case is that of baby Bellagio, a premature infant whose treatment in a neonatal intensive care unit spanned a short, 10-day period. The second case is that of Mr. Cathcart, a 34-year-old man with acute leukemia whose treatment on a medical unit and in an outpatient clinic extended over more than a year. We have deliberately chosen two cases with different age, disease, and treatment characteristics to illustrate the explanatory power of the categories. To protect anonymity, we have altered details about the patients, their caregivers, and the settings.

The case studies invite the reader to experience the world of life–death decision making through the eyes of the fieldworkers. Events are presented in the form of fieldnotes, edited for clarity and continuity. Commentaries are provided to help interpret the action and apply the categories to specific incidents that occur within the case studies.

BABY BELLAGIO

The fieldnotes for baby Bellagio begin on the third day of the infant's life. This baby was born prematurely at 26 weeks gestation and weighed only 950 grams (about two pounds) at birth. Initially, baby Bellagio was not expected to survive more than a few minutes, but, an hour after birth baby Bellagio's heart was still beating strongly and the decision was made to transfer him to a neonatal intensive care unit in another hospital in the city. At Monday morning report, as the fieldnotes begin, the nurses are telling each other about the events of the weekend when baby Bellagio was admitted to the unit.

Day 1

The main focus of conversation this morning in nurses' report was a group of infants who were all described as having questionable neurological status. Baby Bellagio was one of these infants. The nurse giving the report said the physician who made the decision to transfer baby Bellagio to the neonatal intensive care unit (NICU) told her he questioned whether or not he should try to help such a small, premature infant survive. At birth baby Bellagio had been cyanotic with marked indrawing and poor air entry. The Apgar scores were 1 at one minute, and 3 at five minutes. In the end, the attending physician decided to give this baby a chance. Baby Bellagio was transferred by ambulance to the NICU accompanied by a medical student and a nurse. When the baby arrived he had no heart rate, no respirations and no reflexes. According to a nurse who was there, the baby was absolutely black. An NICU resident picked up baby Bellagio and ran up to the NICU where cardiopulmonary resuscitation was begun. After two to three minutes, the infant came around. However, the big question among the nurses is: how long was baby Bellagio without a heart beat? A good deal of concern was expressed about the amount of brain damage that may have occurred during this period.

Commentary The premature birth of baby Bellagio placed the attending physician in a difficult decision-making dilemma. Although he phrased the question in ethical terms—*should* he help the infant survive—the fundamental medical question was *could* he help the infant survive? Even with all possible medical treatment, baby Bellagio might just be too small (that is, too premature) to live. In order to find an answer to both the ethical and medical questions confronting him, it was necessary for the attending physician to make a "getting better–getting worse" calculation. He had to ask himself: what is the evidence to suggest that this infant can survive if given treatment, and what is the evidence to suggest he cannot? In other words, the attending physician needed to make a prediction as to whether baby Bellagio would survive. He would know that the provincial neonatal survival rate for infants weighing less than 1,000 grams at birth was below 20%. On that basis alone, baby Bellagio's chances were not good. He would also know the significance of baby Bellagio's low Apgar scores. (The Apgar scoring system assesses newborn status at birth according to certain objective criteria such as heart rate, color, muscle tone, etc. Scores between 7 and 10 indicate a vigorous infant. Scores of 4 to 6 indicate some compromise, and scores below 3 indicate a severely distressed infant. Apgar scores are highly rated information because of their high correlations with future prognosis. That is, low Apgar scores are associated with poor infant outcomes.) Because the outlook for baby Bellagio was not promising on the basis of these criteria (low neonatal survival rate for infants of baby Bellagio's gestational age and birth weight, and low Apgar scores), the attending physician initially made a "no-aggressive" treatment decision. However, an hour later, he had some counter balancing information that forced him to reconsider this decision: baby Bellagio's heart was continuing to beat strongly. It was at this point that the attending physician decided to give the baby a chance and made what appeared to be an "aggressive treatment" decision. He decided to transport baby Bellagio to a neonatal intensive care unit for specialized treatment. This decision involved a risk–benefit calculation in that the risks of transporting baby Bellagio to the NICU had to be weighed against the benefits. Although the risks of transport were high, baby Bellagio's only hope for survival was to receive the specialized type of care provided by an NICU. A mobility trajectory had to be initiated so baby Bellagio could receive the potential benefits of intensive treatment.

One of the risks associated with a mobility trajectory is that the transitional adjustments necessary to maintain an individual during transport may be inadequate or inappropriate. Baby Bellagio obviously deteriorated during transport to the NICU. At this point, one is forced to question whether or not the transitional adjustments made for baby Bellagio were appropriate, and if not, why not?

Day 1 (continued)

Later in the morning, baby Bellagio was discussed at rounds. The major topic of conversation was the anticipated problem of "weaning" the baby from the respirator. If artificial ventilation continued too long, lung dysplasia might develop. Although there was no firm decision regarding the infant's treatment, the consensus was that baby Bellagio should not be aggressively treated. In other words, the feeling was that the baby "should be left alone."

Commentary More than 70% of infants of baby Bellagio's size and gestational age develop a respiratory condition called respiratory distress syndrome (RDS) or hyaline membrane disease (HMD). Ventilatory assistance by means of a respirator is required for infants such as baby Bellagio whose lungs are immature and who do not have sufficient vigor to breathe on their own. The clinical management of RDS is complex and, while advances in technology have contributed to improved neonatal survival rates, the incidence of complications resulting from the treatment itself has increased. High concentrations of oxygen, prolonged mechanical ventilation, and endotracheal intubation have all been implicated as causes of one of the most common complications of RDS—bronchopulmonary dysplasia. The physicians managing baby Bellagio's care were aware that bronchopulmonary dysplasia was a distinct possibility, but they were caught between "a rock and a hard place." The treatment that kept baby Bellagio alive might eventually contribute to his death. At the same time, they had no option but to continue in the hope that this complication would not develop if they did not treat the infant too aggressively.

Running throughout the conversation was the concern about baby Bellagio's ultimate survival potential, particularly his ability to breath on his own, unassisted by a respirator. Essentially, the physicians were in a "holding pattern," waiting for further information about this potential before deciding to alter their treatment.

Day 1 (continued)

After rounds the physician who had ordered the transfer joined some of the NICU nurses at coffee. He asked the head nurse if the infant was still alive. She replied, "Yes, and I want to see you in the nursery right away." He assured her that he would come as soon as possible.

About 15 minutes later he entered the nursery. There the head nurse confronted him and told him she was "sick and tired" of receiving babies in the condition that baby Bellagio was in when he arrived at the NICU. The physician became agitated and immediately began to explain the position he had been in. He said he was damned if he did and damned if he didn't transfer the infant. He would be accused of being too aggressive if he transferred the baby and of not being aggressive enough if he didn't transfer the baby. He had not expected the infant to survive the transport. He had given orders that the infant was not to be resuscitated if his heart stopped. He wondered why the infant had been resuscitated when it arrived because he had phoned and left a message with the resident that the baby was not to be resuscitated. The nurse commented that residents do not have the authority to make that kind of decision, and that it was a little difficult to make such a decision when an infant arrives at emergency in an ambulance.

After the physician left, the head nurse was asked to explain the physician's reasons for sending baby Bellagio to the NICU. She said at a recent meeting of the morbidity and mortality committee, one of its members had put this physician on the spot for not transferring a similar infant. She said the only reason baby Bellagio was transferred to NICU was that the physician felt he had no alternative in view of this prior confrontation with one of his colleagues.

Commentary This excerpt from the fieldnotes is a clear example of a physician being held accountable for decision making by his colleagues and his attempts to justify his actions. It also illustrates the fact that decisions are not always made solely on the basis of objective clinical criteria. Personal factors may play a major role.

The confrontation between this physician and the head nurse explains why baby Bellagio arrived at the NICU in such poor condition. Although it initially appeared as though an "aggressive treatment" decision had been made by sending baby Bellagio to the NICU, the physician was in reality "waffling." Giving orders not to resuscitate is a "no-aggressive treatment" decision, and is neither congruent nor compatible with the previous decision to transport baby Bellagio to the NICU. Waffling between "aggressive" and "no-aggressive" treatment decisions ultimately resulted in inappropriate transitional adjustments being made during transport. When baby Bellagio had a cardiac arrest, he was not resuscitated even though he was enroute to the most aggressive treatment available. Thus he arrived at the NICU with his already limited potential to respond successfully to such treatment further reduced.

This incident shows just how negative the consequences of "waffling" can be. It also illustrates the potential influence that peer pressure and fear of censure has on the decision making process. Unfortunately, when a physician feels forced into a decision he does not agree with, he may only half-heartedly endorse it. Treatment goals then become blurred, sometimes with disastrous consequences.

Day 1(continued)

Before leaving the unit for the day, the comments in the nursing Kardex regarding baby Bellagio were recorded as follows: "Stress to the mother that the baby will probably not make it. Do not give the mother false hope."

Commentary The nursing Kardex was a flip file of cards for each infant in the NICU. On each infant's card was a special section for recording discussions with the parents and their concerns and wishes regarding treatment. Goals for each infant's care and treatment problems and approaches were also outlined. The nursing Kardex increased the accessibility of information about an infant and family to the nursing staff. By taking a few minutes to look at an infant's card, a nurse could obtain a quick summary of the overall plan of care.

In baby Bellagio's case, the nurses wanted to ensure that his parents received the same prognosis information from all members of the staff. They knew nothing is more distressing to parents than receiving conflicting information about their children. The comments on the Kardex indicate that a "death prediction" had been made, and that the nurses are attempting to prepare baby Bellagio's parents for this eventuality. In so doing, they are controlling the information that baby Bellagio's parents receive.

Day 2

Early this morning one of the night nurses was fixing baby Bellagio's IV. Another nurse arriving for the day shift asked this nurse how the baby was doing. She replied, "Oh, he's doing fine respiratory-wise, but who knows otherwise." Her remark probably meant that the baby's neurological status was still a question mark.

After report, a review of the nursing Kardex and the chart on baby Bellagio revealed an entry since the previous day noting that baby Bellagio was at risk for intraventricular hemorrhage. The parents of baby Bellagio had been in to visit. Apparently, the mother refused to touch the baby and the father would not look at him.

Commentary Intraventricular hemorrhage (bleeding into the brain) is common among very premature infants with severe respiratory disease. Although the exact etiology remains unknown, intraventricular hemorrhage is associated with neonatal hypoxia (shortage of oxygen) and mechanical ventilation. Baby Bellagio was not breathing when he arrived at the NICU and his treatment required a respirator. Therefore, he was a prime candidate for intraventricular hemorrhage. The notation on the chart made such knowledge visible, thereby alerting staff to watch for signs of this complication.

Baby Bellagio was not attractive to look at with his tiny limbs, transparent skin, thin body, and disproportionately large head. He was not most parents' idea of the perfect baby. Surrounded by equipment and engulfed by a maze of tubes and wires, his appearance could easily be frightening to parents. The response of baby Bellagio's parents is typical of that exhibited by parents who are in the initial phase of adaptation to the crisis of premature birth. It should not be confused with rejection of the infant.

Day 3

The report of a chest X-ray taken at 9:00 this morning showed that compared with previous examinations there was lung deterioration. Baby Bellagio had hyaline membrane disease which was worsening. In the afternoon another chest X-ray was taken. Now it was noted that the lungs appear slightly over inflated with the bubbly pattern of pulmonary disease developing. Mention was made of the fact that this may be an indication of bronchopulmonary dysplasia. Still later in the day, another chest X-ray was taken. Again it was noted that the lungs are over inflated and the bubbly pattern was now visible throughout. This time the radiologist had no doubts; he concluded that bronchopulmonary dysplasia was developing with great rapidity.

Commentary These X-ray reports document the progressive deterioration in baby Bellagio's pulmonary status. As such, they constitute highly rated information that can be used for future "getting better–getting worse" calculations. X-ray results are an important component of clinical decision making, whereby subjective clinical impressions of improvement or deterioration can be verified with objective evidence. The physicians' fears have been borne out: baby Bellagio has developed the iatrogenic complication of bronchopulmonary dysplasia.

Day 4

At 7:45 a.m., it was obvious at a glance that this was going to be a busy day. Every space seemed filled with either babies, equipment, or people. The desk was littered with charts and lab reports. No one was standing around waiting for morning report. Everyone was either busy caring for an infant, discussing a case, or charting lab results.

Since the previous day one could see how much this baby had deteriorated. He looked much more emaciated. Little ribs were very visible, as were the bones in the ankles and legs. The baby's color was also worse—a dark, bluish-red—and the face and head seemed to have enlarged, particularly the area around the eyes and the top of the skull, which appeared quite swollen. In addition, the baby's skin was more excoriated and there were large red bleeding patches on the baby's ankles. One of the nurses went to the incubator to chart the IV rate, and said: "This baby's going to heaven today." She noted that the baby was now acidotic.

At that moment, the charge nurse on nights came up and put her hands through the portholes of the incubator to feel the baby's fontanel. She asked the other nurse who had been taking care of the baby about the size of the fontanel—how wide it felt and how boggy she thought the whole area was. The nurse replied that it was very boggy. Asked if she thought baby Bellagio had bled into his brain, the charge nurse said, "Well, that's what we're wondering about."

Commentary Baby Bellagio had been identified as being "at risk" for intraventricular hemorrhage (IVH). The clinical signs of IVH include acidosis, a bulging anterior fontanel, and an abrupt deterioration of the infant's condition. The nurses were aware of the significance of these signs and watched for them. When baby Bellagio deteriorated, became markedly acidotic and developed a bulging fontanel, the nurses based their death prediction on these signs. It is interesting to note that the nurse did not say "the baby is going to die"—death predictions are often cloaked in euphemistic terminology. Neither did they state openly without direct questioning from the fieldworker, the possibility that hemorrhage occurred. They did not have to. The experienced caregiver would understand the significance of the acidosis and the bulging fontanel and what that meant for baby Bellagio. When the nurse told the fieldworker that the baby was acidotic, it was her way of indicating that an IVH had probably occurred. The comment was presented as a rationale for her previous statement that baby Bellagio was "going to heaven." To the uninitiated, however, the connection between the two remarks would have by no means been obvious.

Day 4 (continued)

The head nurse said the baby would be going for a CAT scan to confirm the intraventricular bleed. The nurse said the CAT scan will show with certainty whether or not an infant has had an IVH—"you're not guessing."

Commentary The advent of the CAT scan (computerized axial tomography) has made it possible to accurately diagnose intraventricular hemorrhage. IVH is difficult to diagnose on the basis of clinical signs alone in all but the most severe case. This is a good example of how the availability of the latest technological advances can influence the reliability of the information brought to bear in life–death decision making.

Day 4 (continued)

Later that morning the fieldworker reviewed baby Bellagio's chart. There it was noted that the baby's major problems were acidosis, which was perhaps related to an intracranial hemorrhage, and maintaining adequate nutrition. Baby Bellagio was on total parenteral nutrition (TPN), and the comment was made that it was difficult to keep IV's in a baby this premature. The assessment of the baby at this time was that of a dysmature premie with metabolic acidosis and questionable intracranial hemorrhage secondary to perinatal asphyxia. The plan was to manage the infant conservatively.

Commentary Maintaining adequate nutrition is a major problem in the care of small premature infants. Neurophysiologic immaturity coupled with sickness and debilitation results in poor sucking and uncoordinated swallowing. The danger of vomiting and aspiration precluded oral feeding. Ordinary IV therapy with glucose does not meet the nutritional requirements of these tiny infants. Total parenteral nutrition (TPN) delivers adequate nutrition by the parenteral (intravenous) route. Usually, a mixture of amino acids, glucose, lipids, minerals, and vitamins is infused through a central venous catheter, which is used because of the difficulty in maintaining a peripheral vein site for any length of time. Baby Bellagio had not yet had a central catheter put in, and this concern was being expressed in the chart notes. A decision would have to be made about whether or not this should be done. In the meantime, the plan was to be "conservative," a euphemistic way of saying, "we will wait and see whether this infant has had an IVH before deciding to be more aggressive."

Day 4 (continued)

The fieldworker spoke with the nurse taking care of baby Bellagio and asked her whether the baby was having any spontaneous respirations. She said, "Yes, occasional ones." When asked if she considered this a good sign, she avoided a direct answer by explaining that at this stage infants were really susceptible to brain hemorrhage. Asked if in her experience many babies of this age survive, she thought a moment and then, judging by her hesitation and her answer, it was clear she did not want to reply: "I don't know. I've only been here six months." When pressed for an answer she said: "Well, if they survive the respiratory crisis, then a bleed into the head usually gets them." The fieldworker observed that while the nurse was caring for the baby, she did not talk to him as she did to babies with a better prognosis; her care appeared quite mechanical and detached.

Commentary Although reluctant to admit it, the nurse caring for baby Bellagio clearly did not expect him to survive. Her mechanical, "detached" care was typical of a health professional trying to find protection from the impact of a patient's death through emotional withdrawal from the situation. Such "detachment" is commonly associated with a "death prediction."

Day 4 (continued)

During the morning, baby Bellagio's mother phoned and was told there was no change in her son's condition. The Kardex noted the mother's visit of the previous evening. At that time she said she thought the baby looked better.

Commentary The getting better–getting worse calculation made by this mother conflicted with the assessment of the health professionals. While they were predicting the baby's demise, she thought her baby looked better. The obvious question is: what criteria was the mother using to arrive at her conclusion? Unfortunately, none of the health professionals asked.

Day 5

On arrival the field worker went immediately to the incubator where baby Bellagio had been the previous day and noted that he was still alive. The head nurse came up to say that the results of the CAT scan had been negative. Then she went over to the incubator, addressed the baby first and then the fieldworker: "Well, hello there. Look at him sucking on the endotracheal tube. They put in a central line yesterday."

The fieldworker read the chart and the nurse's report of a negative finding from the CAT scan was confirmed. The chart notes also indicated they were going to discuss how aggressively they planned to manage the baby.

During rounds that morning, the management of baby Bellagio was discussed among the physicians and head nurse. The attending physician commented that since the CAT scan showed there had been no intraventricular bleed, there was no reason to withdraw therapy, and that attempts should be made to wean the baby from the respirator. The head nurse asked if there was anything to indicate that the baby had brain damage. The physician responded by saying, "No, not at all. We'll just have to wait and see." He commented that some nurseries were reporting 40 to 50% survival rates in such infants. However, their nursery could not compare with that. He went on to say that within this 40 to 50% survival rate, a significant number of infants had abnormalities.

At this time another nurse looked at baby Bellagio and commented on his very small size. The head nurse briefly related baby Bellagio's history and mentioned that the baby was doing well respiratory-wise, and that the CAT scan had been negative. She was very enthusiastic in her explanation, and concluded saying, "Oh, he sucks on his endotracheal tube and grabs his hand. He's doing well, the only problem is that period of apnea during transport."

The X-ray report today indicated there was a severe consolidation in both lungs. The chart notes commented that although they planned to manage the infant aggressively for the time being, the X-ray reports indicated broncho-pulmonary dysplasia with a severe form of RDS. The chart also noted that if they establish beyond doubt that the infant has bronchopulmonary dysplasia, they would reevaluate future aggressive treatment.

Commentary The negative CAT scan result was obviously a highly rated piece of information that directly affected clinical decision making. On the basis of this, a decision was made to treat baby Bellagio aggressively and for the first time hopes were raised that this infant just might survive. The CAT scan was the evidence that tipped the balance in favor of continuing aggressive treatment. Had the CAT scan shown blood in the ventricles, it is clear from the physician's comments that his decision would have been different.

The negative CAT scan was obviously as significant for the nurses as it was for the physicians. Their response to baby Bellagio became more optimistic as they began to risk emotional involvement by starting to talk to him in the same way they talked to other infants.

However, the fear of problems remained. Had baby Bellagio suffered brain damage as a result of the apneic episode during transport to the NICU? If baby Bellagio survived, would it be as a normal child? Based on his knowledge of the outcome in similar cases, the physician knew there was a good chance baby Bellagio would have long-term problems. So optimism was tempered with an appreciation for the difficulties that still lay ahead. Baby Bellagio had severe RDS and if he indeed had bronchopulmonary dysplasia, there was little reason to rejoice. The negative CAT scan had only postponed the possibility of a "no-aggressive" treatment decision; it had not ruled it out.

Day 6

The chart notes said baby Bellagio had bronchopulmonary dysplasia with severe RDS. The plan was to continue respiratory treatment. The problems discussed were wasting (loss of 20% of body weight), bronchopulmonary dysplasia, and prematurity with one major setback, that is, cardiac arrest during transfer to the NICU.

Day 7

The plan was to do no further tests or initiate any extraordinary procedures. The situation was discussed with the parents and a decision will be made regarding further management at morning rounds.

Day 8

Respiratory therapy and parenteral nutrition were being maintained, but on the progress sheet was the comment: "supportive treatment only." It was noted in rounds this morning that the parents were not yet ready to make a decision and that the baby will be "kept going for now."

Day 9

All agreed that the situation was now hopeless. The baby's lungs had deteriorated to a point incompatible with life. This was discussed with the parents, who now agreed to discontinue all life support.

Day 10

Baby Bellagio was extubated this morning. He managed to continue breathing for a short period of time before becoming apneic, and died shortly before noon.

Commentary By Day 7 of data collection it became clear that the health professionals caring for baby Bellagio were "giving up." The optimism associated with the negative CAT scan had been short lived, and it was now apparent that there would be no cure for baby Bellagio. He weighed less than 800 grams and his lungs were useless. He could be maintained for a time on his respirator, tubes, and equipment, but the final outcome was inevitable: he would not survive no matter how aggressively he was treated.

Having made a "no-aggressive treatment" decision, the difficult task facing health professionals was helping baby Bellagio's parents reach the same decision. This was done gradually over a period of several days. The parents were not pushed; they were given time. While health professionals were ready to discontinue life support sooner than the parents, they nevertheless maintained baby Bellagio with "supportive treatment" until his parents were able to make that final decision. This is a good example of a sentimental order calculation. Although the health professionals could not help baby Bellagio, they were at least able to give the parents time to accept the inevitability of their son's death.

MR. CATHCART

It was the fourth day of data collection on the medical unit when the fieldworker first heard about Mr. Cathcart. She was trying to get an idea of the routines on the ward, and was sitting with nurses in the conference room after morning coffee. One of them, Mrs. Denver, said they had re-admitted Mr. Cathcart to the ward the previous day; she thought he would be a good patient to follow. She added, "He was diagnosed a few months ago as having acute leukemia, and he's quite bad now. The tragedy is that he found out about this only a month after his marriage." The fieldworker decided to follow Mrs. Denver's advice and read through Mr. Cathcart's chart to find out more about him.

Day 1

Mr. Cathcart had been diagnosed as having acute myelogenous leukemia about six months previously. He was treated aggressively with combined chemotherapy, and the disease was brought under control after two months of hospitalization. But, after only three months at home, the disease spread into his central nervous system forcing his return to the hospital for chemotherapy into his spine and radiation therapy to his head. He was only home a week before he was re-admitted again. Acute myelogenous leukemia—referred to as "AML" by doctors and nurses working in oncology—is the worst kind of leukemia; it tends to strike young adults. Mr. Cathcart had just celebrated his 34th birthday.

After lunch, the fieldworker met Dr. Dennis, the oncologist, to discuss which of his patients to follow for the study. He went over each case, summarizing the medical plan of treatment. But when he got to Mr. Cathcart, he just shook his head and said, "There's not much we are going to be able to do for him."

Commentary From the interactions with Mrs. Denver and Dr. Dennis, it was clear that they both viewed Mr. Cathcart as a "tragic case." From the nurse's standpoint, his social circumstances at time of diagnosis defined the sense of tragedy, while for the physician, it was the lack of treatment options that was troublesome. The initial treatment only worked for three months before the leukemia spread into the nervous system. Both nurse and physician made getting better–getting worse calculations, and had decided that his prognosis was grim.

Day 1 (continued)

At 5:00 p.m. the housestaff gathered in the conference room for their daily chart rounds. They went through the patients on their service one by one, discussing treatment and deciding what orders to write. When they got to Mr. Cathcart, the resident said: "We'll be starting him on chemotherapy tomorrow." At this both of the interns chimed in, saying, "Oh no, we won't." Then one of them explained, "He only has 500 polys and his other counts are very low as well." The resident responded: "Well, is he in his single room yet? I asked them to move him this morning."

Commentary The interns were concerned that the patient's blood components responsible for fighting infection (white blood cells, which include the "polys") and for controlling blood clotting (platelets) were too low to start chemotherapy. The chemotherapy would further reduce these counts, and place him at risk of dying from an infection or hemorrhage. The resident was concerned that the patient was already at risk of serious infection, and for this reason had requested that Mr. Cathcart be moved to a single room. This would allow them to start reverse isolation, a technique to minimize the patient's exposure to the potentially infectious microorganisms in the hospital environment.

Day 1 (continued)

The intern said Mr. Cathcart was not yet in a single room, so reverse isolation could not be started. Apparently, the patient then occupying the only single room on the ward was extremely noisy, and the nurses did not want her moved. The intern was obviously upset, and commented: "It's sad that a man who is so young and 'with it'—I mean he's well aware of what's going on—has to be pushed around like this." The other intern tried to ease the concern saying, "Well, when you're in the hospital you can't always get things exactly the way you'd like to have them." The resident's note in the chart summarizing Mr. Cathcart's current status said: "Getting worse. Most likely causes are nerve root infiltration with leukemia and blood deterioration."

Commentary In this discussion we get an indication of the control that nurses may exert over mobility trajectories. Here they made a "work order calculation," and decided that the noisy patient needed the room more than Mr. Cathcart. Accordingly, the resident's request was not carried out. The housestaff are justifiably upset; they are acutely aware of the risk of infection to Mr. Cathcart as long as he is not on reverse isolation. Here again, we become aware of why Mr. Cathcart is a "tragic case;" he is so young and "with it." The housestaff's frustration is accentuated by the fact that they recognize how quickly this patient is deteriorating.

Day 5

By this day Mr. Cathcart had been transferred to the single room. The ward clerk said the "noisy lady" had been moved out of that room on Friday. She added that Mr. Cathcart really should have had the single room from the time of his admission, but they needed it for this lady so the other patients on the unit could get some sleep.

The chart said Mr. Cathcart was being given a short course of chemotherapy. By mistake, however, he only received half the dose he should have had on Sunday. Mr. Cathcart's white blood cells had dropped considerably and his temperature was elevated. The housestaff still worried about infection.

Commentary For Mr. Cathcart, receiving an underdose could be just as serious as an overdose, because there would then be questions about the adequacy of the trial. That is, if Mr. Cathcart did not respond to the treatment, would it be because his disease was nonresponsive to the drugs, or because the dosage was inadequate? This mistake occurred on the weekend, when staffing and "on call" systems are least adequate.

The housestaff's urgency to get Mr. Cathcart into reverse isolation appears to have been justified because he now seems to be developing an infection. Still, the nursing staff believed that, in the best interests of the other patients, they had no choice but to keep the noisy lady in the single room.

Day 5 (continued)

The nurse caring for Mr. Cathcart said he was walking around, and this would be a good time for the fieldworker to go in to introduce herself.

Mr. Cathcart was a tall, emaciated and bald man who was pacing up and down, stretching his intravenous tubing to its limits as he paced. The label on the IV bottle showed that he was receiving his chemotherapy. The room was bare and dismal—even more so than the other rooms in this old wing of the hospital. The fieldworker introduced herself and the study; he said she could stay and talk. He didn't sit down though, so while he paced, they discussed what had happened to him. He told her he had received chemotherapy three times. The first time he had been able to go home and get back to work; after the second time he was home only a week before the doctors told him his blood counts were bad and re-admitted him; and now this. He also told her about the radiotherapy to his head, which had caused his hair to fall out. He spoke slowly, and would walk silently for several minutes before adding details about his treatment.

The fieldworker asked for his thoughts on these treatments. Was it a natural thing for him to decide to have the therapy? Did he have any questions about his treatment? He replied that he really didn't have any questions. He thought the only thing he could do in the situation was take the treatments.

Mr. Cathcart went on to describe his financial problems. He was diagnosed shortly after his marriage, and had just bought a new house and a new car. He was too sick to move into the new house and his friends had to help. He and his wife had heavy financial obligations, and would be in more difficulty if it were not for his wife's income. He hoped his disability insurance would come through soon.

The fieldworker thanked him for their conversation, and asked if she could return in a few days.

Commentary Mr. Cathcart was obviously content with "provider-con-controlled" decision making. He did not see that he had any option but to accept the treatment prescribed by the physicians. The impact the disease and treatment was having on his personal life was obviously of prime importance. He was no longer able to play the roles of husband and bread-winner as he had intended, and this weighed heavily upon him.

Day 9

The resident said Mr. Cathcart was finished with his chemotherapy, but his problem with nerve root infiltration had not improved. In fact, the pain in his legs was getting worse, and the attending physician had changed his analgesic order from demerol to morphine. The resident added that Mr. Cathcart's counts were very low, with only 600 white blood cells and 22,000 platelets.

Later that morning the nurse gave Mr. Cathcart his new analgesic, intramuscular morphine. He refused, saying he wanted it orally. After all, he said he was already bleeding and had many bruises because of his low platelets. The nurse agreed he might bleed into his muscle after the needle, and made arrangements for oral morphine.

Commentary Although Mr. Cathcart did not influence the design of his therapy, he did exercise veto power over a specific treatment when he knew it would increase his discomfort. Until Mr. Cathcart refused the treatment, neither the physician leaving the order for the intramuscular morphine, nor the nurse implementing the order, remembered that Mr. Cathcart's low platelet counts made such injections risky. Interestingly, Mr. Cathcart was assertive about his treatment with a nurse, whereas he remained essentially passive in his interactions with physicians.

Day 9 (continued)

As the fieldworker left the hospital that evening, she met one of the unit nurses who said how upset she was about Mr. Cathcart. She thought he was getting worse. She said she had a hard time taking care of him because "he's so young." She added, "I've had to reexamine some of my own philosophies since caring for this man."

Commentary This nurse's reaction illustrates the effect a "tragic case" can have on health professionals. Everyone knows Mr. Cathcart's story: he is young, he was diagnosed shortly after being married, and now he's getting worse. The physical and emotional care required by this man has forced the nurse to take a hard look at her own life: if this could happen to Mr. Cathcart, it could happen to her too.

Day 12

On Saturday morning housestaff rounds, it was noted that Mr. Cathcart had gone home on a weekend pass. The intern expressed some surprise that the attending physician had let the patient go when his counts were so low that he required isolation technique. The clinical clerk ventured the opinion that Mr. Cathcart was "going crazy" in the isolation room and needed to get out. The head nurse added that there were probably fewer germs at home than in hospital anyway.

Later, when the attending physician came by, no one questioned Dr. Dennis about his decision to send the patient home for the weekend. The resident said Mr. Cathcart had developed a hematoma on his back, presumably because he had bumped himself and because his low platelet count did not stop the bleeding. Dr. Dennis agreed with the resident's analysis.

At evening rounds, the resident noted that Mr. Cathcart's platelets were down to 4,000. "No wonder he bled into his back." The resident instructed the intern to phone Dr. Dennis to see if he would want to give platelets as soon as the patient returned to the hospital, explaining: "He'll want to give them. You'd better phone him."

Commentary Housestaff generally defer to decisions of the attending physician unless they have a strong, contrary opinion. The decision to send Mr. Cathcart home was not a major one, and so was not questioned. Housestaff also anticipated what a particular attending physician would want done in a specific circumstance, and planned their care accordingly. Again, the patient's blood counts were important indicators in planning treatment.

Day 14

Mr. Cathcart returned to hospital with a low grade fever. Dr. Dennis decided to start him on antibiotics intravenously rather than waiting for his temperature to rise further. His white blood count was only 400.

Commentary The attending physician recognized that for a patient like Mr. Cathcart, an infection could prove fatal if he waited too long to start antibiotics. In this case, the potential benefits of the antibiotics could be lost if they were not started within the appropriate time frame.

Day 14 (continued)

The fieldworker called on Mr. Cathcart. He said he had enjoyed his weekend, but was feeling miserable now. He attributed this to his temperature and the intravenous drugs. He said they also gave him platelets as soon as he returned to hospital and this had stopped the nosebleed he acquired at home.

He talked about his being in the isolation room, and how this affected him: "I know it might bother some people, but I really don't mind." The doctors from the infectious disease service came in, asked him a few questions and left.

Dr. Dennis came in next and examined Mr. Cathcart's chest. Dr. Dennis explained that they had started him on these drugs to lower his temperature and make him "feel better." He added that Mr. Cathcart's blood was low, and they were thinking of giving him a unit of blood. Dr. Dennis then asked if he felt weak. Mr. Cathcart replied: "No, I don't feel any weaker. I just feel worse because of this. . ." pointing to the intravenous. He said he hoped the antibiotics would make him "feel better." Before leaving, Dr. Dennis said he explained the new treatment to Mrs. Cathcart when she phoned him that morning. Before leaving, he tried to reassure Mr. Cathcart: "Well, your platelets are fine. There's no problem there, so don't worry about bleeding. We'll take care of your temperature with the antibiotics, and give you some blood since your hemoglobin's low. Everything's fine." Mr. Cathcart sat silently on his bed as the physician left the room.

Commentary The housestaff's concern about the risks of Mr. Cathcart's weekend at home appeared justified. He developed both infectious and bleeding problems. However, their perception that the reason for Mr. Cathcart's weekend pass was the stress of isolation was not borne out by Mr. Cathcart himself. Why was he sent home with such low counts? Only the attending physician knew for sure, and the housestaff were not asking.

Dr. Dennis obviously tried his best to be optimistic with Mr. Cathcart in spite of the life-threatening nature of his disease and its complications. To do this, the physician focused on the problems caused by the disease rather than on the disease itself. The physician's underlying pessimism is revealed through his choice of the words "feel better" rather than "get better." Both he and Mr. Cathcart knew that the latter was no longer a possibility.

Day 15

Mr. Cathcart said he was feeling much better. His temperature was down, and he thought the drugs were doing him some good. He explained that his financial status was also better now that his disability insurance had come through and he had made some money by selling his snowmobile. He explained: "If I want to go to Skidooing next winter, I'll buy a new one. Even if I go home now, I'd be too weak to use it and I might get a cold."

Day 18

At the evening nurses' report, it was noted that Mr. Cathcart's temperature reached 39° C, and his antibiotic therapy was switched. The day nurse giving the report said that Mr. Cathcart was feeling "blah" all day, but then so was everyone on the unit. The heating system had broken, and everyone was sweltering inside in spite of subzero winter temperatures outside. Just prior to the housestaff's evening chart rounds, the fieldworker discussed Mr. Cathcart with the intern who was pleased that the patient's counts were finally improving, and thought his bone marrow must be recovering from the chemotherapy.

Commentary The antibiotics that had appeared to be fighting Mr. Cathcart's infection were obviously no longer beneficial because his temperature was once again elevated, so a decision was made to switch the therapy. His risk of dying of infection was decreasing as his blood counts recovered after the chemotherapy. However, his life could still depend on the physicians finding the appropriate treatment for his infection.

Day 19

Last evening and night Mr. Cathcart's temperature rose to 39° C again. As soon as the results of his morning blood work came back, the ward clerk brought them into the conference room for the head nurse to see; all the blood counts had improved. The head nurse smiled and said, "Good."

Commentary Mr. Cathcart's blood counts were the most highly rated information in planning treatment, followed closely by his temperature. The blood counts defined his risk of infection and bleeding, as well as for his recovery from the chemotherapy. As a result, blood counts became the most important indicators in getting better–getting worse calculations.

Day 27

When the fieldworker returned to the unit, she learned that Mr. Cathcart was to be discharged; she also asked the oncology resident what the plans were for his care. The resident said Dr. Dennis decided to send the patient home because he was spending so much time alone, and was depressed about his situation. The resident explained Mr. Cathcart was not in bone marrow remission; they had tried every drug available and had only achieved a remission after the first treatment. Therefore, they decided to wait for him to develop new symptoms before treating him further. The resident expressed some doubts about how long Mr. Cathcart would be at home before getting worse.

The resident went on to explain that Mr. Cathcart probably acquired this central nervous system problem with the leukemia because they achieved a first remission. Such first remissions used to be rare in this form of leukemia, but were now becoming more frequent. With this prolonged survival, there was an increased chance of central nervous system involvement.

Commentary The physicians treating Mr. Cathcart were out of treatment options, so they decided to send him home. They hoped he would have some time when his disease remained under control, but were not optimistic that this would be very long. The treatment for this type of leukemia illustrates the risks associated with improvements in treatment; the better the treatment, the longer the survival but the greater the chance of serious disability due to the disease.

Day 77

At evening chart rounds the fieldworker found Mr. Cathcart had been read-mitted. The evening nurse interrupted rounds to ask about Mr. Cathcart's pain medication. The medical student said he had just talked to Dr. Dennis, who wanted Mr. Cathcart to have Brompton's cocktail left at the bedside. The intern suggested the cocktail be given every few hours in a certain dose because it would take awhile for Mr. Cathcart to get used to it. But the medical student insisted that Dr. Dennis wanted the drug left by the bedside so Mr. Cathcart could have as much as he wanted.

After rounds the medical student reported on his conversation with Dr. Dennis. Apparently, they could do no further chemotherapy because the bone marrow simply could not tolerate it. Therefore, all they really had left was pain control. The medical student added, "It makes me mad!" Asked why, he just shrugged his shoulders. "Because he's so young?" the fieldworker asked. He replied, "Yes, and because he was only married three weeks." He said he tried to stay with Mr. Cathcart, leaving himself open in case Mr. Cathcart wanted to discuss the problems he was facing. But Mr. Cathcart had not said much. The student added, "But doing that won't help me treat his disease."

Commentary Mr. Cathcart's readmission signalled a shift from active therapy to palliative or comfort-oriented care, symbolized by the attending physician's order for Brompton' cocktail. He wanted Mr. Cathcart to have unlimited access to this drug, a solution of oral morphine frequently used in treating chronic pain associated with end stage cancer. The young medical student was having a hard time accepting this shift in the goals of therapy, even though he realized there were no other effective options left. Even his attempts to provide some psychological support proved fruitless. Unfortunately, the medical student did not know that Mr. Cathcart's reaction to him was the same as his reaction to all caregivers: passive acceptance of the treatment and of his fate. Basically, the medical student believed you cannot really help a patient unless you can cure the disease.

Day 77 (continued)

Later the head nurse checked through Mr. Cathcart's chart. She said she really noticed how much worse he was since his last admission but she thought he would get some pain relief with the Brompton's cocktail. She added, "But he might get sort of knocked out—it's pretty potent stuff."

Just then a nurse returned from pharmacy with Mr. Cathcart's Brompton's cocktail. The head nurse was about to make up a medication ticket, but looked puzzled when she read the order: "Well, I guess they want it left at his bedside." She shrugged her shoulders, and stared silently at the bottle. Finally, she said, "You know, he could just drink it all at once; he could commit suicide." She asked another nurse to put the bottle in the refrigerator, saying she would ask the resident about the order when he returned to the unit.

Commentary Even experienced physicians may perceive there is little they can do when cure is no longer possible. When Dr. Dennis made the switch to palliative care, he relegated responsibility for deciding the drug dosage to the patient. It was difficult to imagine Dr. Dennis giving Mr. Cathcart the same responsibility for deciding on his chemotherapy dosages.

The nurse's fear about leaving the solution of oral morphine at the bedside was certainly justified. The side effect of drowsiness, which is common with this drug during the first day or two of its administration, could easily lead Mr. Cathcart to forget how much of the drug he had taken and mistakenly overdose himself. In this sense, the risk of treatment could outweigh its benefits. In addition, the nurses were concerned that a young man in Mr. Cathcart's situation—with an increasing number of complications from a fatal disease— might take his life. After all, the nurses were no strangers to euthanasia requests from patients similar to Mr. Cathcart.

Day 81

Over the weekend, there was a consult to the infectious disease service about Mr. Cathcart. The service reported that the patient was not infected at present but they would follow him. The chart noted that the Brompton's cocktail had worked for a couple of days in relieving the patient's pain, but was now no longer providing relief. The patient wanted something stronger, like a needle. Later in the day, the fieldworker noted that the housestaff had left an order for hyperduric morphine.

   Commentary It was not surprising that Mr. Cathcart did not receive sustained relief from the Brompton's cocktail because he received no help in adjusting and regulating the dosage. In this sense, he received an inadequate trial of therapy. However, the trial was not repeated; the treatment modality was switched instead.

Day 82

The head nurse said Mr. Cathcart had taken his Brompton's cocktail over the weekend, but without effect. The physicians had started him on hyperduric morphine, and it was helping to ease the pain but was not entirely effective. The physicians apparently were thinking of trying acupuncture next to relieve his pain. She said the plans were to discharge him home without any treatment because there is nothing left to offer him.

Day 83

The fieldworker talked to Dr. Dennis about the plans for Mr. Cathcart. He said they were thinking about acupuncture for his pain, and as soon as his counts were better they would send him home. Asked whether he had run out of treatment options for Mr. Cathcart he agreed, saying he had given Mr. Cathcart all this intensive treatment without any lasting effect on his disease.

Day 103

The head nurse said Mr. Cathcart was released home a few days previous. Asked whether he had gone home on any treatment she said, "No, just with the morphine." She said they had switched him to the morphine pills when they sent him home, and he was not too happy about that, because he said the pills did not do him much good. She wondered how long he would be at home before returning to hospital.

Commentary Control of symptoms in patients with end stage diseases often require innovative treatment approaches. In this case, Mr. Cathcart's nerve damage was causing intractable pain that the physicians thought might benefit from acupuncture. At least, such treatment would not hurt and it might help. Beyond such palliative care, there were no options left for treating the disease.

Although staff were aware of Mr. Cathcart's pending discharge, appropriate transitional adjustments were not made. He was treated with parenteral morphine until discharge, and then was sent home on the same oral morphine that was previously ineffective in controlling his pain. As far as Mr. Cathcart was concerned, transitional adjustments for his discharge home were woefully inadequate.

Throughout these two hospitalizations, health personnel were consistently pessimistic about the outlook for Mr. Cathcart. They were all convinced what the ultimate outcome would be, and as a result their treatment attempts sometimes appeared half-hearted. When faced with a patient for whom cure is not possible, health professionals are often unable to define alternative goals for treatment. At times, it appeared that the health professionals were so caught up in mourning their own inability to treat the disease, that they forgot Mr. Cathcart was not yet dead and had to continue living with the problems caused by his disease.

Day 298

In the outpatient clinic, the fieldworker was surprised to see Mr. Cathcart's name on the day's list of patients. Dr. Dennis said Mr. Cathcart had been in remission from his leukemia for the past seven months and was now in clinic to receive some immunotherapy.

The fieldworker went in to talk with Mr. Cathcart while he was waiting for his treatment. When she remarked that his last batch of drugs seemed to have worked he replied, "No. They really didn't. They may have helped my leukemia, but they sure didn't help my legs." He said he could not get out and do much walking because his legs still hurt. Asked whether he was surprised that the drugs had helped his leukemia he said, "Well, the most important thing is that I've been able to be at home rather than in the hospital."

He said he had been told why he was getting immunotherapy but he could not remember the details. He agreed to talk again when he returned to clinic the next month.

Commentary Although the health professionals caring for Mr. Cathcart were skeptical about how long he would be able to remain at home, their getting better–getting worse calculations were inaccurate; he had remained at home with only outpatient treatment for seven months. As a result, the physicians renewed their efforts at active treatment.

Even though the short course of chemotherapy was effective in controlling his disease, this was not the most important factor to Mr. Cathcart who was more interested in reducing the problems of living with his disease than in futile attempts at cure. In spite of this, Mr. Cathcart once again passively accepted active treatment, even though it added to his discomfort.

Day 315

The fieldworker learned from the outpatient clinic nurse that Mr. Cathcart was admitted to the hospital. He had phoned the clinic a few days ago to describe his decreasing vision. He came in for an examination and the physician found almost no vision in one eye. Mr. Cathcart returned the next day for a lumbar puncture, which revealed that the leukemia was once again in his central nervous system.

The fieldworker went to the hospital and found that Mr. Cathcart was not on his usual unit because it had been full when he was admitted. When she found him on another unit, the fieldworker introduced herself because she knew he could not recognize her due to his failing vision. He remembered her, and the two sat to talk. He said his sight was not good and that he could not read at all. He looked discouraged as he said this, adding that he had not anticipated this complication. His vision had started to deteriorate about a month previous. He said this was a bad time of year to be in the hospital, just before Christmas, even though his wife had completed all the shopping. He said a neurologist and a radiotherapist were supposed to be seeing him. When asked if that meant more treatments, he said he really didn't know.

He seemed quite drowsy, so the fieldworker asked him if he wanted to be left alone so he could rest. He said no, lying around only made things worse. He said, "It really gets a guy down." So she stayed and they talked about general things for awhile.

Commentary   Mr. Cathcart's depression at this latest in the long string of complications was obvious. The loss of his vision was unanticipated, and the fact that it required his hospitalization just prior to Christmas was an added blow.

Day 316

Dr. Dennis said they were going to irradiate the area behind Mr. Cathcart's eye in order to arrest the process of the leukemia affecting his eye. He added that the existing damage probably could not be reversed, but that they wanted to keep it steady. He said their goal was to give some quality to what life the patient had left. He recognized that reading and watching television were two things Mr. Cathcart could enjoy, because his leg problems limited his mobility. He concluded that the treatment now would be symptomatic, and there would be no further attempts to control the underlying disease.

Commentary Now that Mr. Cathcart's disease has recurred in his central nervous system, he is obviously getting worse. The newly initiated immunotherapy would be discontinued. Once again, the physicians have given up on aggressive treatment. Comfort-oriented care was being attempted, even though the physician recognized such treatment would have limited effectiveness. In Mr. Cathcart's case, the radiotherapy was palliative rather than curative.

Day 336

The head nurse said Mr. Cathcart was dying. He deteriorated rapidly over the holidays, although his vision remained about the same as a result of the radiotherapy. He is getting oral morphine for his pain, but it is not very effective.

Mr. Cathcart seemed much thinner than he was before Christmas. He recognized the fieldworker, and they sat and talked. He was weak, and had a hard time staying awake. When the fieldworker told him she was going away for a couple of weeks, he looked her straight in the eye, and said: "Then I think we'd better say goodbye now." Both knew what he meant. She then told him how much she had appreciated all he had shared over the previous months, and he said gruffly, "Well, thanks for coming in to talk."

DISCUSSION

Although it is true that most life-threatened patients will be cured or at least will have their disease controlled, we deliberately selected two cases with a low probability of cure to illustrate the complexity of life–death decision making. In such cases, many treatment decisions are required and the risks associated with them are significant. Our analysis of the cases of baby Bellagio and Mr. Cathcart demonstrates the usefulness of the categories in explaining complex events. Moreover, we selected these two cases to emphasize that even the most aggressive treatment does not always produce a cure.

Our case studies show that the process and outcomes of treatment are to a large extent determined by the social context within which care occurs. This was true for both baby Bellagio and Mr. Cathcart, although the circumstances were totally different. Each case emphasized that all participants need to understand the influence of the social context on decision making. Without such understanding, health professionals will be less than effective decision makers, and patients and families will lose valuable opportunities to participate in their care.

The issues raised by the cases of baby Bellagio and Mr. Cathcart were typical of those we encountered throughout our fieldwork. First, certain technical knowledge is required to understand events in the treatment of life-threatened patients. While we provided such knowledge in the commentaries, this explanation of events is seldom, if ever, available to patients and families. While health professionals do attempt to explain the disease and planned treatment, they usually do not identify the critical pieces of knowledge and information that patients and families must understand if they are to make sense of ongoing events. Moreover, health professionals tend to communicate in a "shorthand" manner that is usually unintelligible to patients and families.

A second issue raised by our case studies is that the sights and sounds associated with care of the seriously ill can be extremely disturbing. Both baby Bellagio and Mr. Cathcart were physically "ravaged" by their disease and treatment and such unpleasant visual images evoke strong emotional responses in both family members and caregivers. Any analysis of life–death decisions that ignores this neglects an important factor in the human response to treatment decisions.

Third, it should be clear from the case studies that there is never just one, overall treatment decision. Rather, care of the seriously ill patient requires a series of decisions. When a patient is critically ill, the intent of therapy can change rapidly, depending on the patient's response. The pattern of care may follow an up-and-down course, in which optimism suddenly gives way to pessimism, or vice versa. These sudden shifts in outlook are emotionally draining for all participants.

Fourth, it is obvious that modern treatment for life-threatening illnesses involves considerable risk. If seriously ill patients want the benefits of treatment, they also must accept certain unavoidable risks. The complexity of health technology is such that patients may die from complications of treatment rather than the disease.

Finally, it should be clear that health professionals are committed to providing the most comprehensive treatment they can for life-threatening illnesses. Regardless of this commitment, they sometimes make mistakes. However, even when health professionals provide flawless care, there are limits to existing knowledge and technology. Unless health care consumers recognize such limits, they will place unrealistic expectations on health professionals and be unprepared for the harsh reality that cure is not always possible.

11

IMPLICATIONS
AND RECOMMENDATIONS

In this final chapter we examine the implications of our findings for consumers, health professionals, and the health care system. These implications pinpoint changes that are needed to improve the overall quality of life-death decision making. We have formulated a series of recommendations that culminate in an audit procedure that can be used to judge the quality of life-death decision making within any setting. We believe the implementation of such audits will convince health professionals of the need to pursue the more general and far ranging recommendations we have outlined.

In keeping with our approach throughout this book, our recommendations do not emerge from any particular ethical or moral perspective. Rather, we are convinced a pragmatic approach to improving care for the seriously ill is needed to avoid the dehumanization that will inevitably accompany the increasing reliance on technological intervention. We believe our recommendations have the potential to initiate a reassessment of current health care practices. We hope such reassessment becomes the stimulus for a more collaborative approach between consumers and health professionals as they confront this difficult field of health care.

HEALTH CARE ORGANIZATION

Our description of health care organization revealed five major problem areas: inaccessibility of medical rounds to non-physicians; diffusion of responsibility for patient care among physicians; the lack of transitional spaces within the health care system; limited availability of health personnel in specific circumstances; and inappropriate health care policies. We explore potential solutions within each of these problem areas.

While the structure of medical rounds provides a natural forum for decision making, the basic issue is how to make them more accessible to non-physicians. To influence decision making, all participants with relevant information need to be present at rounds. Yet nurses—who act as storehouses of much relevant data—and families—who possess the "lifestyle" information needed in decision making—are usually not involved in the process of "rounding." The seriously ill patient may be too sick to state a viewpoint, and it is usually too difficult for families to plan their lives around the medical schedules of rounds. The result is that information deemed important by the patient or family may not be brought forward at the time when critical treatment decisions are being made. The current structure of rounds, in which only physicians are included, systematically omits information that patients and families view as relevant in planning their health care.

One solution is to designate a health professional to systematically represent the views of the patient and family during rounds. In other words, rounds could not proceed without the presence of this health professional in much the same manner that rounds cannot now proceed without the presence of the attending physician. Such a role could, for example, be assumed by a nurse within each critical care setting. The process of eliciting and representing the views of seriously ill patients has traditional roots in nursing and is advocated as an important role in the profession today. Nurses are already responsible for relaying information important to the treatment plan, but at present such information is usually medical in nature. Moreover, patients and families will often share information with nurses that they are less likely to mention to physicians because they think doctors are too busy to be bothered with their day-to-day concerns.

However, if such a role were to be assumed by nurses, changes in nursing education would have to occur. The ability to present information concisely and to argue persuasively for a viewpoint is emphasized in medical education, and such skills would be required by the health professional selected to be the patient/family representative at rounds. Nurses will need specific educational preparation for this role if they are to become effective participants in life–death decision making. Such preparation could be incorporated into the final electives found in the senior year of most undergraduate nursing programs.

For the structure of rounds to become more flexible and open to information input by non-physicians, other changes will have to occur. Medical education must then emphasize the importance of such information in addition to the traditional reliance on test results and physical findings. The concept that the decision making process is incomplete without considering the patient and family's viewpoint will need to be developed early during medical education and emphasized in subsequent clinical assignments. Only through such a shift in perspective will the input of a health professional designated to represent patient/family views have any influence on treatment decisions.

With the proliferation of medical subspecialites, diffusion of responsibility for decision making will become an increasing problem. As more and more physicians are consulted during the decision making process, the opportunities for waffling will increase, with the consequence that no definitive treatment decisions may be made at all. Waffling is particularly risky when the time frame for decision making is short and the patient's survival depends on an appropriate treatment decision being made quickly. The health care system must develop structures to minimize this risk. The task of coordinating the activities of all the health professionals involved in a complex case is important and is often assumed by a medical resident or primary nurse. This coordinating activity is critical to the effectiveness of life–death decision making, and needs to be recognized formally within the health care system.

We have illustrated the problems that can occur when an appropriate space for treating the life-threatened patient is not available within the system. However, the obvious solution—to increase the amount of high technology space for care of such patients—is not a viable one. Rather, we need to rethink the approach to clinical space within the health care system, with more emphasis on transitional space. Most seriously ill patients are initially treated in a high technology environment, but where they move after this phase depends on whether they get better or worse. If they are getting better, they need to move through spaces that are progressively less technological until they return home. If they are getting worse, they similarly need to move into low technology environments once a no-aggressive treatment decision has been made. For example, if death is imminent but the patient still requires intensive nursing care, an intermediate care area attached to the intensive care unit would be an appropriate space. At present, many high technology spaces are occupied inappropriately by patients who no longer benefit from them.

The increased use of the home as a place to die has important implications for health professionals. Physicians caring for patients at home must make house calls, yet their day-to-day work is usually structured such that these visits must be made after all their other responsibilities have been fulfilled. The system needs to recognize the importance of physicians being available to make house calls to dying patients. Similarly, the legal system needs more flexible rules about who can pronounce death when a terminally-ill patient chooses to die at home. The specter of having a recently deceased love one resuscitated by ambulance or emergency room staff should not have to be witnessed by families who have chosen to care for the dying person at home. If the physician cannot come to the home at the time of the death to sign the death certificate, the visiting nurse who has been involved in the case should be able to pronounce death.

The limited availability of health personnel on evenings, nights, weekends, and holidays can produce problems for the life-threatened patient. If the onsite decision maker—for example, a nurse or intern—is only permitted to make "wait-and-see" decisions, the initiation of treatment may be delayed beyond the optimum time frame. Our description indicates that health professionals often put off important treatment decisions when the attending physician is absent. The onsite decision maker should have both the authority and responsibility to proceed with treatment if the time frame is narrow and the attending physician not available. This implies that nurses should have additional education to assume such responsibility in settings where physicians do not provide 24 hour coverage for seriously ill patients. Evaluation of the processes of treatment decision making within a clinical setting using the standardized audit procedure we will describe later could lead to revised staffing patterns and better treatment outcomes for patients.

While there has been much emphasis on the patient's right to consent to treatment, the fact remains that most hospitalized patients will be resuscitated whether they view such treatment as appropriate or not. Changing the resuscitation routine to an individually planned trial would remove a source of controversy in the care of dying patients. Such a change would imply that resuscitation orders and their consequences would have to be discussed with each patient and family entering the hospital in order to ascertain their wishes. The positive consequences of such dialogue would be twofold. Health professionals would become comfortable in discussing life–death issues on a regular basis, and the issue of appropriate treatment for serious illness would be consistently brought to the attention of consumers. The change of resuscitation treatment from a routine trial to an individually planned trial is long overdue and deserves support from the legal system.

TECHNOLOGY AND TRIALS

One of the major problems in health care is that a shift from curative to palliative care does not always occur when cure or control of disease is no longer possible. Our description suggests there are several reasons why it is so difficult to abandon aggressive treatment in favor of "comfort care only." Belief in the curative powers of modern technology is deeply rooted. If one treatment approach does not produce a positive response, then perhaps the next one will, especially if new technology can be incorporated into the trial. This way of thinking leads to every known option being tried, even though the last one implemented usually has only a slim chance of producing any effect on the disease process. The implementation of progressively less effective trials postpones the shift to treatment aimed solely at promoting comfort. The extent to which curative trials are pursued may be more dependent on the number of innovative approaches known to the practitioner than on the patient's response to treatment.

In this often played scenario of diminishing returns, the troubling issue is: at what point should the shift to comfort-oriented care be made? In response, we make several observations. First, while the exact percent chance of response to a curative trial is discussed in the physician group at rounds, precise figures are usually not offered or requested when the physician outlines to the patient and family the next treatment approach that could be tried. Rather, general terminology is used: "It's less effective than the last treatment we gave, but I think it's worth a try." As a result, patients and their families do not have the information they require to decide how worthwhile it is to continue attempts at cure.

The rapidity with which the diminishing returns actually "diminish" may also influence their perspective. For example, if successive trials offer an 80% chance of a cure and then only a 20% chance of temporary response, the patient's choice about whether or not to continue aggressive treatment may be different than if he is offered a series of trials that promise an 80, 70, 60%, etc., chance of cure. Each of us might ponder what our response would be to these alternative scenarios. However, in a real situation we would probably not be given these figures, and we might well be too sick or too frightened to ask for them. As long as health care consumers are shielded and shield themselves from this type of information they will not be able to decide at what point the shift to palliative care is appropriate.

Another reason why curative trials continue beyond the point where they produce results is that the intent of the trial may not be clear. For example, after a no-aggressive treatment decision has been made, complications may nonetheless be aggressively treated. That is, although efforts to cure the disease are abandoned (usually because everything has been tried and nothing has worked), attempts are made to correct every complication. The refrain, "at least he died with his electrolytes normal," is not so far from the truth. This lack of clarity about the overall intent of treatment can result in dying patients being maintained in critical care areas.

The decision to abandon aggressive treatment and switch to comfort care can be difficult to implement if an appropriate space is not available for the patient within the system. The lack of a "place to die" is one of the most striking characteristics of the modern tertiary care hospital. Transitional spaces designed for the care of the seriously ill or stabilized patient who is no longer receiving curative trials are generally not available. As a result, the dying patient must be cared for in strongly curative, highly technological environments. As we have noted, when technology is available, it tends to be used. The dying patient cared for on a critical care unit is at greater risk of suffering the consequences of waffling than is the dying patient being cared for in a palliative care unit.

Even if a transitional space designed for comfort-oriented care is available, it may not be used. Transfer to such a unit externalizes the no-aggressive treatment decision, whereas maintaining the patient in the cure-oriented environment enables the patient, family, and health professionals to maintain the pretense that curative treatment is continuing. For example, even simple interventions such as daily blood tests have symbolic meaning long after their results cease to be used in designing treatment. The act of discontinuing such interventions conveys a clear message, one that health personnel may not wish to communicate, and the patient and his family may not wish to hear.

While health professionals receive extensive educational preparation in how to help seriously ill patients get better, they have little or no training about comforting the patient who is getting worse. The concept that there is nothing left to do for a patient for whom aggressive treatment has been discontinued is still prevalent. For example, recent advances in management of pain and other distressing symptoms are not integral parts of most undergraduate medical and nursing programs. It is not surprising that today's practitioners think there is nothing they can do for a patient if they cannot cure his disease. The curative emphasis in the undergraduate programs of most health professionals fosters this attitude and tends to perpetuate the lack of transitional spaces for the dying. If palliative treatment is not recognized as a valid specialty, it is unlikely that space for this care will be developed within an already competitive and overcrowded health care system.

The reasons why the transition from curative treatment to palliative care does not always occur are many and complicated. More precision in decision making would be one approach to encouraging the implementation of comfort-oriented care when cure or control of the disease is no longer possible. First, precise information regarding the known effectiveness of the treatment being offered should be communicated to the patients and families who must consent to treatment. Second, the overall intent of treatment should be clearly communicated to all participants by the designated decision maker. Third, once a decision is made to stop curative treatment, the patient should be protected from reinstitution of curative attempts. Adherence to these three principles of good decision making would clarify much about care-giving intents and actions, which are often left implicit. Finally, when the health professional decides to ignore these principles he or she should at least ask, "Who am I really treating here? Myself, or the patient?"

While we are not optimistic that the issues we have raised will be quickly addressed, there are nonetheless things that consumers can do to soften the impact of the curative trial. First, it is imperative that informed consumers become involved in the planning meetings during which standardized pre-planned trials are formulated. Questions regarding the treatment's toxicity and lifestyle impact can then be raised from the perspective of those receiving rather than those administering the treatment. In this way the treatment plan could be designed in recognition of both the need to increase survival and to maintain a reasonable quality of existence during treatment. Even those patients who automatically consent to treatment would benefit from such activity.

Second, consumers can request individually planned trials. As our description indicates, treatment is often adjusted in response to such requests, but it cannot be altered if health professionals are not aware of individual circumstances. Our recommendation to designate one nurse to bring patient and family perspectives to rounds would enable even reticent consumers to benefit from individualized treatment. Commitment to curative therapy does not imply surrender of all control over the decision making process, as we shall discuss in the next section.

CONTROL AND PARTICIPATION IN DECISION MAKING

At present, patients and families exercise little, if any, control over final decisions about treatment. Our description indicates that many seriously ill patients will not participate in decision making even when they are encouraged to do so. There is a certain mystique implicit in the total surrender of life-death decisions to the "experts." Yet the truth is that giving away all responsibility for treatment decisions does not guarantee a cure. Treatments are imperfect, and any patient may end up on the wrong end of the percentages, even when cure rates are favorable. While physicians are among the first to admit that their decision making is fallible and responses to treatment uncertain, many patients believe they will be cured provided they follow the prescribed treatment.

Our description indicates that reality contradicts this widespread belief. Even if the patient is cured or the disease brought under control, the chance of experiencing some iatrogenic complication or long-term disability is high. Disappointment and anger with the physician who was supposed to guarantee a cure with minimal discomfort can lead patients to rely on folk remedies instead.

The fact is that treatment for most life-threatening illnesses is long and arduous. Accepting the treatment plan usually involves a commitment to considerable discomfort and disruption in lifestyle, and may even involve accepting the possibility of dying from the side effects of treatment. Accepting treatment also means that the seriously ill patient may endure risk and discomfort but still die of the disease. Given this reality, it is surprising that more patients and families do not wish to participate in decisions about their health care. However, fear of discussing such realities is no doubt a major force inhibiting health care consumers from evidencing more interest in critical treatment decisions.

Several strategies could be implemented to inform consumers about their options should they become seriously ill. Large scale consumer awareness programs could use television or radio messages to educate the public about general issues such as resuscitation. Consumer education programs for specified populations in the community could address more specific issues such as the importance of family members discussing among themselves their wishes should they become seriously ill. If consumers are to affect the design of treatment, they must understand what options they have.

While we have described four patterns of control over treatment decisions, it seems that joint control offers the greatest possibility for positive outcomes. When the physician is the sole decision maker, patients may resent their lack of control, especially when treatment does not deliver what was promised. When the patient or family exerts final control over treatment, they may later regret their choices or feel the health care system has failed them. Joint control offers the potential for avoiding these problems as well as several others. For example, patients would not have to withhold consent for a treatment with which they disagreed because consent would be mutually negotiated. When the patient, or family, and the physician share the burden of responsibility for selecting the final course of treatment, litigation is less likely. Litigation concerns may lead to "safe" decisions, rather than the best decision for the seriously ill patient. Problems with noncompliance should be reduced because there would be a greater commitment to the selected course of action on the part of the patient and family. Finally, patients, their families, and physicians would not be able to avoid communication about short and long term prognosis since this information is essential to the decision making process.

The shift to joint control as the model of choice for control over decision making would have implications for both education and practice. Strategies such as family conferences could be systematically implemented to foster joint discussion of treatment approaches. Within particular subspecialty areas, groups of physicians could discuss and formulate approaches to joint decision making that recognize the special concerns of treating life-threatened patients in their clinical area. Subspecialist groups in which the model of joint decision making is well established could then serve as models for undergraduate students, because it is difficult for young health professionals to assume a model of practice unless they understand what it looks like and how it works.

While the joint approach to control over decision making represents a goal for the future, there are still patients who wish to play no role in treatment decisions and those who wish to make all their own decisions. At present perhaps the best the health care system can offer is to ensure that the patient's control preference is realized. While the patients who wished only to follow physician's treatment plans experienced few difficulties in the past, legal requirements for informed consent now mean that they must at least listen to explanations about treatment even if little of this information is actually remembered. In contrast, patients who wish to select their own treatment from the range of options available will probably encounter considerable opposition if it conflicts with the treatment preferred by the attending physician. Such patients risk being abandoned both by their caregivers and the health care system. Movement toward the model of joint control over decision making would provide a more flexible approach to formulating effective treatment plans that are acceptable to all participants.

DECISION MAKING

Without knowledge and information, neither health professionals nor patients and their families are able to participate effectively in treatment decision making. However, health professionals usually have access to this knowledge and information while consumers do not. As our description illustrates, health professionals control the flow of information and can effectively exclude patient and family from decisions by failing to communicate vital data. Such failures to communicate are often not intentional. Rather, the fast-moving nature of this field of health care is such that information changes so quickly that it may become obsolete even before it can be used in planning treatment. In addition, the amount of information generated can overwhelm even the medical team attempting to decide which data is relevant to diagnosis and treatment. Absorption in the day-to-day difficulties of providing care to seriously ill patients is more often the reason patients and families are not informed about ongoing test results and treatment options, rather than any deliberate attempt to withhold information.

Nonetheless, lack of information sharing with patients and families represents a major problem in this field of health care. When they first develop a serious illness, most consumers do not even know what questions to ask to elicit the data most relevant to treatment decision making. For each major life-threatening illness, consumer groups could formulate a series of general questions to guide lay people during their initial interactions with health professionals. Simple questions such as the following could be formulated to assist a patient who suspects that his diagnosis is cancer: "What are the results of my biopsy? Does that mean it's cancer? Has it spread?" Later, another set of questions might be used: "What are my treatment options? Are there any other options you have not told me about? Could you tell me how successful each of these options are? Could you tell me what the side effects of each treatment are? How will each of these treatments interfere with my day-to-day life?" While such questions are simple and straightforward, they are usually not asked. As a result, the information received by the patient and family depends on what information health professionals choose to share. Unless consumers become more assertive and consistent in their questioning, their information base will be incomplete and their opportunities to influunce the design of treatment very limited. While the designated decision maker should take responsibility for reviewing relevant test results and treatment options with patients and families, the more consumers expect this to occur and make their expectations known, the more likely that such information sharing will become the norm.

While patients and families may receive varying amounts of information about their disease and its treatment, they usually begin with a knowledge base drawn largely from experience. This knowledge base will influence their perception of specific pieces of information and their resultant decisions about participation in the planned treatment. As our description indicates, apparently inexplicable behavior of patients and families may emanate from previous experiences that family members or friends have had with a similar disease or treatment plan. Health professionals should systematically elicit this experiential knowledge during their initial assessment. Unless attempts are made to clarify similarities and differences between the present illness and the one experienced by a friend or family member, it is obvious that consumers will use the only knowledge base they have to guide their decisions.

While information about the patient's previous lifestyle is highly rated in decision making for the adult, it is often not readily available when treatment decisions are made. Our recommendation that a health professional be designated to represent the views of the patient and family at rounds would provide a means of ensuring that lifestyle information is both available and accessible. Similar strategies need to be implemented within each clinical setting to ensure that other important medical information is available when decisions have to be made. Evaluation of a number of clinical settings using the audit procedure to be described could identify the most effective of these strategies. As our description illustrates, limited availability or accessibility of information during the appropriate time frame can have drastic consequences for the life-threatened patient.

Risk–benefit calculations remain the most frequent approach to life–death decision making. Assessment of the risks and benefits attached to various treatment options is usually accomplished by physicians talking among themselves and weighing relevant test results and physical findings in the light of current knowledge and research data. As our description indicates, the selection of the "best" treatment options may be relatively simple or extremely complex. But, even when the calculation is relatively simple, the process of decision making may not be communicated to the patient and family. Why is the treatment option favored by the attending physician superior to the other options considered? What are its chances of working? What is the nature and frequency of the attendant risks? While the favored treatment option is usually explained, the answers to such questions may not be volunteered or sought by the seriously ill patient and family. Once again, the overwhelming and frightening nature of the illness inspires the health professional to be protective, while the patient and family are awed into reticence.

Whether consumers should be privy to the entire process of risk–benefit calculations is a difficult issue. On the one hand, the volume of knowledge and information weighed during complicated risk–benefit calculations is sometimes overwhelming even for health professionals so that sharing such detailed considerations with an already stressed patient and family becomes formidable. On the other hand, straightforward explanations about the primary risks and benefits of the attending physician's treatment of choice as well as the next best alternative would provide the patient with the basis for giving a truly informed consent and for correcting the risk–benefit analysis by supplying additional data. If the patient wished to delegate responsibility for final selection of treatment to the physician, at least he would have heard about the second alternative. Assuming there is more than one treatment option, consistently presenting at least the top two ranking options could foster development of the joint control model of decision making. Perhaps the most difficult task facing health professionals today is how to present complex, technological information in a straightforward manner. Testing different approaches for the presentation of risk–benefit calculations may help us understand what is best from the patient and family perspective.

Our description indicates some physicians are reluctant to pursue high risk-high benefit treatment. Patients may not be referred for risky treatments and as a result they are denied the potential benefits of such therapy. Continuing education for community physicians should be aimed at demystifying high risk-high benefit treatments so there is greater understanding of the specific circumstances under which such treatment is justified. Seriously ill patients may become resentful if they discover they have not even been offered a potentially beneficial treatment because the physician was not willing to accept the attendant risks.

The getting better–getting worse calculation raises similar considerations. The indicators used by health professionals to make such judgements are usually invisible to families, and confusion and mistrust results unless these indicators are made explicit. Eliciting the indicators being used by patients and families to judge deterioration or improvement should also be part of the ongoing assessment. When these indicators are explicit, differences in the judgement process can be recognized and discussed. When they remain implicit, treatment recommendations may be viewed as inappropriate, unacceptable, and misunderstood.

There will be times when risk–benefit and getting better–getting worse calculations are suspended in favor of the work order calculation. Given the current structure of health care, such decisions are sometimes necessary to maintain the functioning of units that provide care to the seriously ill. However, each time such a judgement is made, the fact that it is being made should be explicit to all and the potential negative consequences for the patient should be outlined. If this approach were adopted, work order calculations could be restricted to those that benefit institutional functioning without increasing risk to the patient. Because nurses are often involved in such calculations, the implications of making such judgements if they result in negative outcomes for the patient should be explored by professional nursing organizations.

Many physicians experience difficulty when confronted with a multiple-persons calculation. The process of weighing the benefits of a particular treatment or service for a group of patients and then deciding who is benefiting least is not easy. Yet restrictions on resources as health care funding becomes limited increases the need for such decision making. In addition to the traditional emphasis on treatment decision making in the one-to-one doctor-patient relationship, medical education needs to address the issue of how to allocate scarce resources within patient groups. Such training is particularly important in the postgraduate programs for critical care services.

A sentimental order calculation usually occurs when some participants have difficulty accepting a no-aggressive treatment decision. Staff may not be ready to give up because they have worked so hard and so long to help the patient get better. The family as a whole or one family member may not be quite ready to accept the inevitable. In either circumstance, the patient's life is maintained until they are convinced aggressive treatment should be withdrawn. In these circumstances, the fact that a sentimental order calculation is being made should be clarified. In addition, whose sentimental order is being maintained—that of the staff or or family—should be explicit. Such clarity in decision making is necessary if staff responsible for implementing care, particularly housestaff and nurses, are to understand the ongoing plans for treatment.

Quality of life calculations tend to be used more by patients and families than health professionals. However, as we have noted, risk–benefit calculations may include quality of life factors as specific risks or benefits. The type of communication we have recommended for risk–benefit calculations would enable patients and families to revise or add those risks and benefits that are really quality of life issues. Health professionals are unlikely to be responsive to general arguments that "life is no longer worth living." But quality of life factors included in a risk–benefit calculation appeals to their "scientific" approach and can tip the balance for or against treatment. Further, our recommendation to designate a health professional to represent the views of patients and families at rounds would ensure that ongoing risk–benefit calculations are formulated using quality of life factors. Patients and families must discuss among themselves what aspects of life makes it worth living. They will then be in a better position to influence those aspects of decision making that have a profound effect on their overall quality of existence.

Our general recommendation is to increase both the precision and visibility of decision making. Obviously, the type of decision making process or processes being used should be specified. Our description provides a typology to permit such specification. Second, decision making should be carried out within an appropriate time frame. Such a time frame is defined as the maximum time that can be used to gather knowledge without seriously jeopardizing the patient's survival. Of course, time frames will vary, but the consequences of making a decision too late can be drastic for the seriously ill patient. For example, repeated wait-and-see decisions may result in no definitive treatment until it is too late for the patient to benefit. Third, the current informal reliance on skilled decision makers should be extended and formalized within the health care system. These physicians can act as role models for decision making beyond the confines of their own subspecialties. Fourth, each clinical setting should conduct periodic reviews of its decision making processes using the criteria we will outline. Finally, systematic evaluation of the outcomes of all decision making processes—rather than only those that result in death of the patient— should also be conducted regularly. At such reviews, the distinction between preventable and unpreventable iatrogenic complications should be made so that better strategies for reducing preventable complications can be formulated.

Increased precision in decision making may be most evident in the way it reduces waffling and its negative results even though it may or may not change the outcome. The experienced decision maker recognizes that the best decision given the amount of information and knowledge available within the optimum time frame may also be the wrong decision. Alternatively, a good outcome may be due more to good luck than good management. The goal should be to optimize both the quality of decisions and the quality of outcomes.

IMPACT

The impact of participating in life–death decision making can be devastating for patients, families, and health professionals. The recommendations we have suggested thus far should help reduce some of the confusion that occurs in this fast-moving and crisis-ridden environment. For example, if waffling decreases because it is clear which decision making process is being used, nurses are less likely to be forced into explaining inconsistent treatment plans to families. Patients and families are more likely to feel satisfied with the health care being provided if their information is valued and if they have an opportunity to influence treatment decisions. Physicians will benefit when decision processes are explicit and can share responsibility for difficult treatment decisions. Changing the care of life-threatened patients in the manner we have outlined will probably have the greatest effect in reducing the stress on all involved.

However, the effects of caring for the seriously ill are such that specific supportive measures are also required. The undergraduate education of both nurses and physicians needs to include classroom content and clinical practice in communicating with life-threatened patients and their families, and how to provide comfort care after a no-aggressive treatment decision has been made. Under the guidance of competent role models, young health professionals should be able to practice the specific responsibilities they will be expected to assume on graduation. For medical students, issues such as how to deliver bad news and how to provide pain management for the dying should be addressed. Nursing students should learn how to design nursing care and provide psychological support to reduce the helplessness experienced by life-threatened patients and families. It is not fair to thrust young health professionals into situations where they must provide specialized and stressful care without any specific preparation for their task. Worse, negative first experiences may cause them to avoid interaction with the seriously ill. Undergraduate education for the health professions in general should be redesigned so that feelings of competence rather than fear are encouraged in our young practitioners. Fostering such competence will necessarily lead to improved collaboration with patients and families, better decision making, and reduced psychological stress on all participants. In this way, education provides a key for the future improvement of all aspects of life–death decision making.

Within high stress environments such as critical care units, it should be recognized that life-threatened patients and their families need additional psychological support by building it into the formal structure; for example, a designated person—social worker or chaplain—trained and competent to provide such support. As a caregiver who does not provide treatment, such a person can provide a neutral and nonjudgemental approach to the problem facing adults in much the same way that the child support worker does in a pediatric setting. In addition, this support person could provide bereavement followup to families as well as support to staff members who are troubled by the death of a patient. These important functions cannot usually be assumed by staff within the setting because of their already heavy responsibilities and close involvement in the treatment program. The need for adult-to-adult psychological support in this field of health care is acute.

AUDIT PROCEDURE FOR LIFE–DEATH DECISIONS

At present, examination of the efficacy of life–death decision making is restricted to the outcome evaluations that usually occur during mortality rounds. Such evaluations are retrospective rather than prospective in nature, and the processes by which decisions were made for all life-threatened patients over a specific time period are not systematically scrutinized. Our description of current practice suggests that such scrutiny is indeed warranted.

We will outline a series of criteria that could be used to audit the effectiveness of life–death decision making in any clinical setting. We suggest that the audit team include: (1) a physician in the clinical specialty of the majority of the physicians within the setting and who is viewed by colleagues as a skilled decision maker, (2) a nurse who is a clinical specialist in the setting to be audited, (3) a health administrator with experience in designing and administering the overall functioning of a unit such as the one under audit, and (4) an informed consumer who is involved in issues related to the care of seriously ill patients. Such a team could be assembled by any agency responsible for funding health care.

For such an audit to be effective, it should be prospective in nature. That is, a random sample of a specified number of cases admitted to the unit over a specific time period should be followed from admission. The criteria we outline could be used as a basis for developing reliable checklists by which trained observers/interviewers could gather quantitative data for evaluation by the audit team. In this way, specific areas of strength and weakness in decision making for life-threatened patients could be identified, and specific recommendations formulated for each clinical setting audited. If a large number of clinical settings are audited in this manner, specific deficiencies within a geographic area (i.e., a state) could be identified and programs designed to remedy such deficiencies.

An important question about such an audits is: "Would health professionals change their behavior if they knew they were being audited?" Perhaps. But our experience in participant observation indicates that health professionals have a difficult time maintaining behavior that is unusual for them. An adjustment time must be allowed for staff to become accustomed to the presence of the observer/interviewer. Since health professionals are by and large committed to improving care for the seriously ill patient, the audit procedure might provide a welcome opportunity for them to examine their own decision making processes.

The criteria that follow emerge directly out of our description of current health care practice as it effects the life-threatened patient. Taken as a whole, they provide a practical means for evaluating the day-to-day process of life-death decision making within specific health care settings. However, they may also be useful for professional self-evaluation; for example, a physician may wish to rate himself on the extent to which he met these criteria in treating his last case. Similarly, the life-threatened patient or family may use these criteria to examine the adequacy of health care they are currently receiving. These criteria also provide a way for both lay people and health professionals to communicate more effectively with each other. The more specific we become in identifying problems within this field of health care, the greater our chances of being able to do something about them.

CRITERIA FOR EVALUATING LIFE–DEATH DECISIONS

1. Is someone (preferably the attending physician) clearly designated as having final responsibility for treatment decisions?
2. Does this designated decision maker accept and exercise this responsibility?
3. Is the designated decision maker the focus of incoming information?

4. Does the designated decision maker accept responsibility for communicating with patient, family, and other health professionals about how decisions are made and when to expect definitive treatment decisions?
5. Alternately, has the designated decision maker formally delegated these communication tasks?
6. Is there a decision maker designated to make definitive treatment decisions in the clinical setting 24 hours a day, seven days a week?
7. Is lifestyle information and the experiential knowledge base of the patient/family considered during decision making?
8. Is the patient/family allowed to express a preference for the degree of control they desire over treatment decisions?
9. Are relevant test results and treatment plans shared with the family as an important part of the decision making process?
10. Is the type of decision process used clearly specified?
11. Are high risk–high benefit treatments systematically avoided?
12. Are the indicators used in getting better–getting worse calculations explicit?
13. How do work order calculations affect the patient?
14. Are all health professionals aware when a sentimental order calculation is being made and why?
15. Does the decision process demonstrate sensitivity to quality of life factors?
16. Are decisions made within the optimum time frame?
17. Is the intent of curative or palliative treatment clearly indicated?
18. Is the decision process subject to periodic internal review?
19. Are clear distinctions made between preventable and unpreventable iatrogenic complications?
20. Are all treatment outcomes of life–death decision making systematically evaluated?
21. Is there a designated support person available within the clinical setting?

Of course, it would be impossible for any clinical setting to meet all of these criteria for all cases sampled. Changes in staffing, a particularly complex case, and many other factors operate to produce uneven performance on these criteria even in a setting with a reputation for delivering excellent care.

Our intent is that these criteria can be used for self-evaluation by health professionals, patients, and families, and by the staff of clinical units, as well as for the systematic auditing of units within a geographic area. While the former procedures are important to maintaining excellent care within a unit, the latter is essential if we are to recognize systematic deficiencies within the health care system. At present, such deficiencies gain attention when unusual cases are reported in the media or brought to the courts, or as a result of a single patient or family writing about their experiences. This way of identifying deficiencies in life–death decision making is clearly unsystematic and biased, yet it is such cases that mold the public's perceptions about the care they can expect when they become seriously ill. The only way to influence such perceptions in a positive way is to provide systematic and unbiased evaluations of the current state of affairs. If health professionals demonstrate a commitment to pursue such evaluations, consumers can have confidence that the first step toward improving this field of health care has been taken.

APPENDIX
Research Methods

THE METHODS

The processes of life-death decision making were studied using an inductive research approach known as participant observation, or fieldwork. This research included such specific strategies as directly observing the events surrounding life-death decisions: interviewing people who had participated in or had witnessed these events; and examining documents such as patients' medical records and written health care policies. The descriptive data were collected in 14 health care settings in Manitoba. These data were systematically categorized using content analysis. A comprehensive description of what happens when treatment decisions are made for patients with life-threatening illnesses was subsequently developed.

Approach to the Study

In any research endeavor, the way investigators think about the problem under study influences the methods they select to collect and analyze the data. In our research, we adopted a general perspective called "symbolic interactionism." This approach to the study of human behavior rests on three premises. First, human beings act toward things on the basis of the meanings these things have for them. Second, meanings arise from social interaction; and third, meanings are modified through an interpretive process used by the person in dealing with the things encountered.

Take, for example, the case of the physician in an intensive care unit who, while observing a young man unconscious after a motorcycle accident, makes the statement: "What a waste." This physician is responding to the situation on the basis of its meaning for him. The meaning he attaches to the situation has been formed by social interactions with others, perhaps by observing other young people who die after such accidents, or perhaps by arguing with a son who wants to buy a motorcycle. The physician's previous experiences have then influenced his interpretation of the present situation.

As a research perspective, symbolic interactionism calls for a naturalistic approach to the empirical world. We selected this approach because we believed that a close examination of the real world of life–death decision making was needed. While much had been said about what "should" be done to change this world, there was no systematic description of what actually happens. Without improved understanding, recommendations for change could either prove fruitless or potentially dangerous to the quality of health care.

Settings

Data were collected in 14 health care settings in Manitoba from February 1975, through September 1978. The settings for data collection were:

1. Two adult medical-surgical units
2. Two adult intensive care units
3. Two adult outpatient clinics
4. Homes of patients in the urban community through a visiting nurse service
5. An adult palliative care unit
6. A northern nursing station
7. A labor and delivery unit
8. Two neonatal intensive care units
9. A pediatric intensive care unit
10. A pediatric medical unit

All of the institutionally based settings were in either of the two large teaching hospitals in Winnipeg, a city of almost 600,000 people.

Methods of Data Collection

A combination of research approaches generally described as "field methods" were used in the data collection. The four field methods used most frequently were: (1) direct observation of events, (2) interviewing participants during events, or (3) informants who had witnessed events, and (4) document analysis. At the onset of data collection in each setting, more time was spent observing and analyzing documents than interviewing. This approach was necessary to become familiar with the settings and to enable study participants to get used to the presence of an observer.

Direct observations were made under a variety of conditions. Sometimes we happened to be present when significant events were occurring. More often, however, we had to discover when and where decisions were usually made and then be present to observe at those times and places. For example, optimum observation times were attending physician or housestaff rounds, medical conferences where treatment decisions were made, and nurses' reports. At other times, direct observations involved following people during part or all of their daily work. Sometimes it was most effective to remain at the bedside of a patient or at a key position on the unit, especially if a significant event was ongoing. Decisions were made daily to select the optimal timing for observations in order to yield the best data.

Interviews of participants and informants were most often in the form of brief conversations carried on at opportune times during daily activities. For example, we frequently asked questions about the nature or intent of treatment plans during medical rounds. At other times, more lengthy conversations occurred informally, such as when a participant explained the approach to decision making with a particular patient or group of patients. Such conversations often occurred in hallways or while enroute from one site of care to another. Frequently, arrangements were made to interview medical personnel, patients, or families. Key personnel such as medical directors, head nurses, or administrative personnel were interviewed to better understand life–death decisions in their environment. Patients and families were interviewed to ascertain their understanding of the ongoing treatment. Informant interviews helped provide information about events we had not witnessed.

A wide variety of documents were analyzed for the study. Whenever available, the patient's medical record was consulted, and information was extracted and recorded. Among other documents used as sources of data were: hospital policy statements, unit policy statements, statements of medical privileges, forms for recording clinical data or treatment plans, hospital newsletters, and research protocols. These documents were usually essential to understand how the setting functioned and therefore came to our attention during the process of data collection.

Other sources of data used by the investigators included the medical literature as well as papers and opinions delivered at medical conferences. These sources provided information about the North American medical context within which the Manitoba data could be interpreted. For example, results of studies used by Manitoba practitioners to guide their decisions became sources of data for this study.

We realized our presence did change behavior in certain respects. Some participants were initially anxious about being observed, but their anxiety decreased as they became used to our presence. In some units, physicians tended to think "aloud" more than they had previously. In other words, participants tried to make the data more accessible. They were more likely to explain the reasoning behind a decision or their reactions to a particular situation becuase they knew it would be of interest to us. The process of data collection necessarily sensitized many of the participants to the issues and their behavior in the life–death decision process. The extent to which these subtle changes affected the reliability of our data is unknown.

Confidentiality of Data

Several measures were implemented to protect the rights of subjects and to ensure anonymity and confidentiality of data. Consent for participation of health personnel was negotiated in group meetings before observation. All persons who did not wish to participate in the study were excluded from both observations and interviewing.

A short, standard explanation of the study was used to negotiate consent from patients and families. Because the information we were seeking related to treatment patients were receiving, they were often willing and able to talk about their experiences. The advice of the nursing staff was invaluable in timing the approaches for such interviews. We were keenly aware of the high anxiety these patients and families were experiencing, and in many cases deferred interviews until a stressful situation had passed or did not seek an interview at all if the situation continued to be stressful. While it might be argued that valuable data were missed by this conservative approach, we had no desire to place additional stress on life-threatened patients or their families. Indeed, to adopt too aggressive a stance would probably have jeopardized the relationships we had established with health personnel.

No written consents were obtained from participants in this study. Negotiated verbal consents are the usual approach in field studies because of the impracticality of obtaining written consents from every person observed. This is particularly true in large institutions where many people pass through a setting in a single day. However, the absence of written consent forms did not change our responsibility for obtaining informed consent from participants.

Specific measures have been taken to ensure anonymity and confidentiality of the field data. Initially, code numbers were assigned to all persons observed or interviewed. The manner in which incidents from the fieldnotes are reported were designed to protect anonymity. Pseudonyms or general terms such as "the patient" or "the nurse" were used in illustrations from the fieldnotes. Highly identifying incidents have not been used as illustrations, and some details have been omitted or changed to preclude identification of participants in the study.

Data Analysis

The constant comparative method of content analysis described by Glaser and Strauss (1967) was used in this study. In this method, each incident or event in the fieldnotes is analyzed to identify its essential content. At the onset of the study, we made lists of the essential content of incidents. After sorting items on these lists into groups, a title was assigned to summarize the common theme in each group. For example, one of the categories identified early in the study was called "measurement of deterioration or improvement in condition."

Once some initial categories were identified, constant comparison of incidents could proceed. In other words, while each new incident was still examined for its essential content, it was also compared with all other incidents. We could then determine whether the incident in question was the same as, or different from, other incidents in a category. If it was the same, the incident was coded into that category. If it was different in content, it was compared to incidents already coded into other categories. If the incident did not fit into any of the categories, the nature of the incident was noted and set aside for future reference.

Whenever possible, the names of the emerging categories were abstracted from the language used by participants in the study. For example, one process of decision making, the "getting better–getting worse" calculation, was derived from statements of health personnel and families such as, "Is he any better today?" or "I think he's getting worse because. . ." Other categories did not lend themselves to such characterization and so were assigned titles by the investigators.

THE EXPERIENCE

The process of data collection for this study immersed us in an unfamiliar environment that was fast-moving, crisis-ridden, stressful, and sometimes confusing. As we attempted to comprehend the world of life–death decisions, we became sensitized to rapid changes in the social processes we were observing. As we listened and tried to understand, we developed increasing empathy for the dilemmas faced by many of the participants. Inevitably, we experienced some of the same emotions and reactions as the people we observed.

Decisions During Data Collection

A central responsibility of any field researcher is the day-to-day decision making of where and when to collect data. The selection of situations for observation and interviewing was often conditioned by events, but decisions to follow particular situations in more depth was at our discretion. Each situation had to be assessed for its potential to contribute to a systematic description of life–death decision making. The time required to track down various participants and arrange interviews was considerable, so the appropriate selection of situations for further data collection was critical. In an important sense, we had to acquire some of the skills of a detective, learning which "leads" to follow in order to acquire the most useful information.

An important aspect of these daily decisions was the selection of strategies to facilitate data collection. The emotional intensity of some events was a significant factor influencing such decisions. We had to decide what type of questions might elicit the most information, and when to ask those questions. In most instances, questions were best asked after a crisis situation had been resolved. However, even in stressful situations, we had to acquire enough information to understand what we were observing. In these cases, questions were kept brief and to the point. At times we had to decide if our presence would create additional stress; if this was the case, we withdrew and then returned later to gather information. Data collection was a process of involvement in and withdrawal from the world of life–death decision making. The appropriate choices of when to go and when to stay were critical in terms of developing our description and maintaining relations in the field.

Difficult Situations in the Field

During field research, there are always moments that stand out from the usual process of data collection. Such situations are probably well remembered because they required quick thinking and challenged our personal resources. In one such incident, we were observing on a medical unit and noted that an elderly woman whose condition fluctuated from week to week always had a pink tag on her nursing record. After several weeks, plans were announced for this patient's discharge, yet the pink tag remained in place. We were intrigued. At this point, we decided to find out what the pink tag meant, and asked the attending physician only to discover that he was also unaware of the meaning of the pink tag. However, our question prompted him to find out that the pink tag was the symbol for "no resuscitation," and as a result, he took immediate action.

> The physician said the pink tag should be removed because the patient was much better. Much to the surprise and dismay of the fieldworker, he called the head nurse and told her to remove the pink tag from the patient's nursing record. The fieldworker then explained to the head nurse that she had only asked about the tag because she thought the patient was going to be discharged. The head nurse was upset and said: "You realize this means the nurses will go ahead and resuscitate the patient if something happens on evenings or nights." The doctor

assented, and said if the patient did get worse, she would be reassessed then. The head nurse was obviously quite angry; she told the field-worker that the nurses would now have no choice but to resuscitate this patient and implied this was all the fieldworker's fault for bringing the issue to the attention of the physician.

In another difficult situation, we were required to make a quick decision about a family member's need for information.

After making some notes, the fieldworker came back to the labor and delivery area to see if the patient who had gone for X-ray pelvimetry had returned. By the hustle and bustle in her room, she could see something was going on. Suddenly, the resident burst out of the room and asked the head nurse to get the patient's obstetrician on the telephone. Then the anesthesiologist came out and also tried to call the patient's obstetrician on another telephone. Soon the nurse came out with the laboring woman on a stretcher and wheeled her down the hall to the delivery room. The patient's husband, who by this time had wrapped himself around the fieldworker, kept asking what was going on. What were they doing? Were they going to do a caesarean section? He knew she was not ready to deliver normally. At this point the fieldworker was in somewhat of a dilemma; she felt this was a good example of lack of information-sharing with the husband on the part of the staff, and that this was what she was supposed to be observing. Yet, on humanitarian grounds, she did not feel she could allow the poor man to suffer any longer with the anxiety of not knowing what was going to happen to his wife. The fieldworker then told him that his wife was going to have a caesarean section.

Both of these incidents illustrate the difficult situations we encountered. The emotional intensity surrounding the phenomena being studied left us open to blame if we made a social error. Similarly, the fast-moving nature of events forced us to make quick decisions about when it was appropriate to move out of the observer-interviewer role. The psychological stress we experienced in these situations was significant, so it was fortunate that such events were rare.

Personal Impact of the Field Experience

Both researchers tried to prepare themselves psychologically for the process of collecting data for this study. Both were aware that issues of death and dying would be discussed by participants. Both had personal and educational experiences such that these topics were not frightening to them. Nonetheless, the intensity of some of the situations we encountered was unexpected and left vivid impressions.

Perhaps the most personally disturbing events were those where patients were disfigured by their disease or treatment. One of the authors had nightmares after seeing a patient turn a hideous shade of green after going into renal failure and retaining a test dye. The other was disturbed after viewing a baby with massive skin necrosis. These images were hard to erase. We can only speculate what effect they must have had on family members.

The other situations that have left enduring memories are those that filled us with sadness for the participants. The emotional pain endured by some family members was so clearly illustrated that at times we were profoundly moved by our experiences.

> *The father entered the nursery to see his baby. The attending physician asked for his home telephone number, and said to the father: "There's nothing more to say, really. We can just wait and see what happens." After the father bent over and looked at his baby, tears filled his eyes and he walked toward the door of the unit. He tore off a wad of paper towel from the sink at the door as he left the room. The father came back to the nursery about 15 minutes later. He had obviously been crying because his eyes were red and swollen, but he put on a nursery gown, washed his hands and went back to his baby's incubator. He stood there for a long time, holding one of the baby's hands and stroking the baby's head. It was an extremely moving experience to see this huge man reduced to tears by a 1,600 gram infant. . . . He then took off the gown and moved to the other side of the incubator where he stood peering through the incubator at the baby's face for a long time before leaving.*

In some of the incidents, we were inspired by the emotional courage of participants, or by their skills and sensitivity in the management of difficult situations. Such events were uplifting because they demonstrated the depth of human experience and quality of health care that is in fact possible. We learned a great deal from the participants in this study, both professionally and personally. However, if asked whether we would do it again, our answer would be uncertain. The physical and emotional stress of collecting the data for this study was considerable, and perhaps it was better that we did not fully appreciate this when we started.

BIBLIOGRAPHY

Aries, P. (1981). *The hour of our death.* New York: Vintage.

Benoliel, J. Q. (Ed.). (1982). *Death education for the health professional.* Toronto: McGraw-Hill International.

Bluebond-Langner, M. (1978). *The private worlds of dying children.* Princeton, NJ: Princeton University Press.

Bosk, C. L. (1979). *Forgive and remember: Managing medical failure.* Chicago: University of Chicago Press.

Bunker, J. P., Barnes, B. A., & Mosteller, F. (Eds.). (1977). *Costs, risks and benefits of surgery.* New York: Oxford University Press.

Cassileth, B. R. (Ed.). (1979). *The cancer patient: Social and medical aspects of care.* Philadelphia: Lea & Febiger.

Corr, C. A., & Corr, D. M. (Eds.). (1983). *Hospice Care: Principles and practice.* New York: Springer Publishing.

Crane, D. (1975). *The sanctity of social life: Physicians' treatment of crticially ill patients.* New York: Russell Sage Foundation.

Feifel, H. (1977). *New meanings of death.* New York: McGraw-Hill.

Glaser, B. G., & Strauss, A. L. (1967). *The discovery of grounded theory: Strategies for qualitative research.* Chicago: Aldine-Atherton.

INDEX